A PLANT POWERED APPROACH TO PROSTATE CANCER

A PLANT POWERED APPROACH TO PROSTATE CANCER

BRUCE MYLREA
WITH MINDY MYLREA

COPYRIGHT

© 2020 by Bruce Mylrea – All Rights Reserved

No part of this book may be copied or reproduced in any form without permission in writing from the publisher, except by a reviewer who may quote brief passages for review purposes. For permission requests, send an e-mail to the address shown below:

Info@onedaytowellness.org

DISCLAIMER

This book is not intended as a substitute for the medical advice of physicians. The reader should regularly consult a physician in matters relating to his/her health and particularly with respect to any symptoms that may require diagnosis or medical attention.

REVIEWS

Prostate cancer is one of the most common cancers in men, but that doesn't mean steps can't be taken to lower your risk. That's where nutrition comes in. A plant-based diet not only provides protection against the disease; breakthrough research shows that it can slow or even halt its progression. In this powerful book, Bruce shares his inspiring journey along with everything you need to know to regain your health.

Neal D. Barnard, MD, FACC
Adjunct Professor, George Washington University
School of Medicine
President, Physicians Committee

This book a must-read for anyone touched by prostate cancer. Bruce reveals with honesty and humor how he leveraged his knowledge of, and passion for, plant-based nutrition, mindfulness, and personal behavioral change strategies not only to help heal himself but also to shine a light of wisdom and hope for others.

Ocean Robbins
CEO, Food Revolution Network
Author, 31-Day Food Revolution

What a refreshing, honest account! The author and his wife, Mindy, use everyday language to describe his journey with cancer. He lets it all out—whatever he thinks, with additional, care-giving comments from Mindy. Bruce reveals the tight linear connection between long-term dietary patterns and cancer development, then goes on to outline how we can leverage simple behavior change strategies to substantially improve cancer outcomes.

T Colin Campbell, PhD
Jacob Gould Schurman Professor
Emeritus of Nutritional Biochemistry
Cornell University

Bruce details his remarkable journey in managing his life with a prostate cancer diagnosis. I was especially impressed with the level of engagement that Bruce made with the research community in order to ensure the accuracy of his writing.

Theodore M. Brasky, Ph.D.
Research Assistant Professor,
Dept. Internal Medicine
Ohio State University Comprehensive
Cancer Center

ARE YOU READY to take back your POWER? Bruce's inspiring story will GET YOU THERE!

I've health coached hundreds of men over a decade now, and they need this book NOW more than ever!

This book is a quick guide for any man that is dealing with Prostate Cancer! It's also a great resource for *all* Health Practitioners to share with their patients!

Michelle Joy Kramer
Board Certified Health Coach, CHHC, AADP
MichelleJoyKramer.com

DEDICATION

This book is dedicated to the two million-plus men who walk in my shoes—men diagnosed with prostate cancer who don't want this diagnosis to be an end or the beginning of an end. So they take action. They find a way to make a prostate cancer diagnosis a new beginning that promises good things to come. And good things do come. I'll show you how I did it.

EPIGRAPH

I choose to be happy.

— Bruce Mylrea

PREFACE

I have never written a book before but I was compelled to write this one for two reasons:

1. I had to get it off my chest.
2. Through no fault of their own, most men diagnosed with Prostate Cancer (PC) are simply unaware of the power of diet and nutrition. I'm in a position to help.

I DO NOT have ANY financial stake in any food, supplement, or pharmaceutical company. My wife's and my non-profit, One Day to Wellness, explicitly does NOT accept any financial support or contribution from these industries. We are simply a force for good. I am not a doctor or a scientist, but I have done my homework on the subject matter that follows, and I strongly encourage you to do the same. I have included an extensive NONSPONSORED resource section at the end of this book. Please use them! They are all FREE!

Part One of this book is a raw summary beginning with my cancer diagnosis nine years ago, followed by the emotional and physical journey since that day. The only way I could do this was to lay everything out chronologically and then do a deeper dive into critical turning points for me personally as they unfolded over the last decade. My goal in doing this is to help you not make the same mistakes that I did when I received a positive PC diagnosis and to hopefully provide you with tools to avoid the pitfalls that men recently diagnosed with PC fall into.

Part Two is a deeper dive into the science and research on why we get so much PC in the US and the industrialized world and how we can use pure unbiased science to help make critical decisions that all men diagnosed with PC have to make.

I have also included a substantial glossary of terms at the end of the book to help with understanding acronyms and definitions. I have also included a resource section with links to great organizations that are focused on evidence-based research without industry influence. Use it—Everything is FREE!

I want to be very clear—I am not proposing that eating a plant-based diet will cure your PC. I AM suggesting that making this change could be one of the most powerful weapons you have in improving your odds of a healthy long-term outcome and feeling vital and energetic along the way. And just as important, a plant-based diet will mitigate or reduce the horrible side effects of standard cancer care.

Scientific research on nutrition as it relates to disease is very difficult. It's never perfect, there is never enough money or time, and researchers have financial interests that can be difficult to trace (on purpose). But even with all the problems and issues, the overwhelming amount of evidence clearly suggests that consuming a plant-based diet is the optimum way to eat if you have PC—or any other chronic illness for that matter.

I am a passionate proponent of eating a plant-based diet because it has completely turned my life around for the better, and I have seen it do the same for scores of other men. The proof is in the pudding. It works.

DON'T FEAR CHANGE—EMBRACE IT. NOW!

ACKNOWLEDGMENTS

I want to thank my wife, Mindy, who came up with this whole idea of me writing a book and made sure I completed it. I live for her and my three sons, Drew, Chris, and Casey.

I want to thank my three sons: Drew, Chris, and Casey, who have stood by me and have always been there for me during my lowest lows and hopefully some of the highest highs.

I want to thank my dad who has always been there for me during this cancer journey as well as the rest of my life.

I thank Dr. T. Colin Campbell for writing *The China Study*. Reading that book was the seminal event in my plant-based journey.

I want to give a special thanks to Dr. Michael Greger who, over the last several years, has helped to guide our non-profit mission One Day to Wellness.

I also want to thank Dr.'s Abrams, Campbell, Barnard, Saxe, Klaper, McDougall, Greger, and Goldhamer for their generous support, time, and perspectives which they have given me in writing this book. I'd take any one of them as my doctor in a heartbeat.

Thanks to Lauren Katz for designing the colorful cover of this book and Grace Michael for her editing magic.

Thanks to Eliud Sibour and his transcription company, Transcriptioncentral.com, in Uganda.

I also want to thank my best friend, Jeff Llewellyn, and his wife, Chris, for all of their help and emotional support for this effort.

CONTENTS

Introduction 1
PART 1 15
   Chapter 1 Who Am I? 17
   Chapter 2 Why Don't We Know 21
   Chapter 3 The Day that Changed My
       Life 29
   Chapter 4 How Did I Get Here? 33
   Chapter 5 Turning Points 41
   Chapter 6 Working for Myself 47
   Chapter 7 Finding Nutritional Research
       and Discovering the Truth 51
   Chapter 8 This Is THE Definition of a
       Turning Point—Eat the Food! 57
   Chapter 9 The Diagnosis 61
   Chapter 10 Surgery and Radiation—
       January 2012 67
   Chapter 11 My First Breakdown in
       NYC 2013 73
   Chapter 12 More Docs and the Beach
       House – Spring of 2013 79
   Chapter 13 Alternative Treatments 83

Chapter 14 The Book, *Fear: Essential Wisdom for Getting Through the Storm,* and the Beginning of My Meditation Practice 87

Chapter 15 I Love Martinis!................................93

Chapter 16 Searching for the Right Team..103

Chapter 17 Therapy—Cannabis 111

Chapter 18 SEX and Intimacy............................123

Chapter 19 WFPB Diet = No OIL.....................127

Chapter 20 Finding MY Team 131

Chapter 21 Find Your Purpose...........................135

Chapter 22 Italy and Fasting 139

Chapter 23 But First More Tests 143

Chapter 24 Breakfast with Dr. Greger at IDEA in July 2017 and the Wellness Wagon 151

Chapter 25 TrueNorth Fasting Adventure September 2018 159

Chapter 26 Breakdown #2..................................165

Chapter 27 I Chose to Be Happy.......................171

PART 2 177

Chapter 28 Digging Deeper 179

Chapter 29 Who Gets Prostate Cancer and Why?.....................................189

Chapter 30 Cancer and Obesity..........................199

Chapter 31 Clinical Trials 203
Chapter 32 Eating Patterns Around the Globe 217
Chapter 33 It's the Food 223
Chapter 34 Plant Oils—The Food Fat Connection 253
Chapter 35 What Do I Eat? 259
Chapter 36 Turning Points— Intermittent Fasting and Intact Grains 265
Chapter 37 Going Forward 277
Chapter 38 What I Do Every day 281
Epilogue 287
Glossary of Terms and Acronyms 291
Educational and Recipe Resources 307
References 309
PART ONE 309
PART TWO 313
About the Author 339
Also Available on Amazon Mindy's Book 341
REVIEWS 341

INTRODUCTION

Write What You Know.

—Mark Twain

My name is Bruce Mylrea; I am 62, and I have advanced prostate cancer (APC). This is my story.

Following is my journey, struggles, successes, and choices which I have made, both good and bad, since I received the diagnosis of having APC. What follows is painful, raw, and real. Why am I telling you about my experience? Because my goal in writing this book is to help other men dealing with the same emotional rollercoaster ride I have been on for the past nine years. I know now what I didn't know when I was diagnosed with APC, and I wish I had someone like me to guide me—someone who navigated the path and could guide me with all the resources available. What I have learned is that your medical team can only do so much. And what they don't know can actually cause you more harm than good. Incorporating nutrition, stress reduction, exercise, mindfulness, and allopathic care allows you to play this awful game with the full deck of cards you need to have at the table.

After being diagnosed with PC, many men play all their cards in their doctor's office. They do not take it upon themselves to seek out all the additional options available that their oncologist might not be aware of. I would have been one of those men but wasn't because I studied extensively, researched, and then made the changes that I did. If I hadn't done these things, I probably wouldn't be here writing this book in an effort to help you.

I know how difficult it can be to begin a radical behavior change process in the midst of what is probably the most difficult time in your life learning that you have PC. I was diagnosed with APC at age 53, a much younger age than most men, and I have spent the last nine years dealing with the American medical system. I have personally witnessed and experienced a stunning lack of knowledge among those in the medical system, and at times, even denial of the proven, measurable benefits of the importance of diet and lifestyle changes in order to, first of all, NOT GET PROSTATE CANCER, but also as an adjuvant treatment of the disease. My observation is that most men after diagnosis still do not grasp the vital importance of changing their behavior, especially as it relates to food, stress management, and lifestyle. And why would they if their doctor has no training in nutrition or alternative therapies and only offer standard or experimental allopathic western medical treatment?

Many men with prostate cancer are also dealing with other chronic conditions such as diabetes, high blood pressure, and obesity. We now know that the majority of chronic conditions experienced in this country can be drastically reduced or even eliminated with diet and lifestyle. And unlike taking drugs to suppress the symptoms, dietary interventions can actually treat the root cause of what is going on, and all of the side effects of diet and lifestyle changes are POSITIVE!

When was the last time your doctor gave you a prescription and told you, "When you start to take this drug, your blood pressure will normalize, your cholesterol will drop, and your triglycerides will drop as well. You will have more energy, sleep better, improve your sexual stamina, and have no side effects." There was no last time that you heard this, was there? But hearing this is available to you NOW! Where/how? Through this book and the things I will share with you.

I needed medical experts to guide me in the current oncological medical world. I bumbled around trying to find the right medical team, but there was no way of knowing who that might be, so my advice to you is to pick a team of medical experts that you trust and are comfortable with. Each team has essentially the same knowledge, but with different perspectives. So, it is an extremely difficult task to find the right team, and you will need to do your homework. It is not my intention to give advice on what the best medical treatments for PC are, nor is it intended to provide specific guidance on what your oncological team specializes in. I am sharing my experience on how I have navigated the frustrating cancer medical system. What this book will provide is the most current research and science to date on what we men can do to take control of our health and improve our outcomes through nutrition, stress reduction techniques, exercise, and mindfulness.

Regardless of your diagnosis, stage, and predicted outcome, this is the most important thing you need to understand: Only *YOU* are in charge of your health. Not your urologist, radiologist, or oncologist. It's just going to be YOU rolling into the operating room with the robots (been there). It's only going to be YOU on the radiation table being physically adjusted for getting zapped (been there a few times too). It will only be YOU ingesting insanely expensive pills that have side effect lists as long as a legal pad (been there too).

It's YOU, and you have way more control over your health and outcome than you probably ever imagined. However, this power and control that can change your life for the better will only manifest when you are willing to open your mind to new research not only in medicine but also in nutrition and lifestyle changes.

You can turn your life around and live a fulfilled life even after receiving a prostate cancer (or advanced prostate cancer) diagnosis. I did. I'm doing it. I can't say that it has been easy, but looking back, all the challenges have provided opportunities for growth for me. I know my story is just one of millions, and disease affects all men differently at different stages, but I want to propose

Introduction

to you right now that if you can embrace a few new basic principles of living and the changing of behavior that comes along with it, this tragic diagnosis can become a catalyst of change. In my case it was a major change, but change that has improved my overall outlook and perceived quality of life.

Regardless of the traditional medical path you take, and I will share mine in the pages of this book, we now have good scientific proof of the highest mechanistic quality (meaning that we can identify a direct link between the food we eat and disease outcomes), that changing your diet along with a few other lifestyle modifications can be one of the best, and in some cases, the most powerful tools we have in our battle with prostate cancer. There is a very good chance that you may have never even heard of this information. There is a reason why: Money. Remember this every time you watch the news on TV and are bombarded by pharmaceutical advertisements touting drug treatments from cancer to diabetes. The vast majority of these drugs *only treat symptoms,* not the root cause of the (usually chronic, self-inflicted) problem. There are massive amounts of money in selling drugs to a fearful, uninformed public. THERE IS NO MONEY IN TELLING PEOPLE TO EAT MORE FRUITS, VEGETABLES, GRAINS, AND LEGUMES.

Despite my having prostate cancer, I have learned to live and thrive through behavioral change, nutrition, mindfulness and meditation, good sleep, and letting go of emotional baggage. Included in each section of this book is research, additional reading resources, and doctors and organizations that treat the whole patient and not just the isolated disease.

As part of my preparation in writing this book, I was fortunate enough to personally interview some of the greatest thought leaders, doctors, and scientists in the world on nutrition and cancer. When pertinent, I provide an "expert analysis" on specific subjects of concern or controversy so we can hear directly from the best minds on the subject. They are as follows:

Neal Barnard, MD, FACC, is an Adjunct Associate Professor of Medicine at the George Washington University School of Medicine in Washington, D.C., and President of the Physicians Committee for Responsible Medicine.

Dr. Barnard has led numerous research studies investigating the effects of diet on diabetes, body weight, and chronic pain, including a groundbreaking study of dietary interventions in type 2 diabetes, funded by the National Institutes of Health, that paved the way for viewing type 2 diabetes as a potentially reversible condition for many patients. Dr. Barnard has authored more than 90 scientific publications and 20 books for medical and lay readers, and is the Editor-in-Chief of the *Nutrition Guide for Clinicians,* a textbook made available to all US medical students.

As president of the Physicians Committee, Dr. Barnard leads programs advocating for preventive medicine, good nutrition, and higher ethical standards in research. His research contributed to the acceptance of plant-based diets in the "Dietary Guidelines for Americans." In 2015, he was named a Fellow of the American College of Cardiology. In 2016, he founded the Barnard Medical Center in Washington, D.C., as a model for making nutrition a routine part of all medical care.

Dr. Barnard received his MD degree at the George Washington University School of Medicine and completed his residency at the same institution.

~ ~ ~

Donald Abrams, MD, is an oncologist at the UCSF Osher Center for Integrative Medicine.

Dr. Abrams provides integrative medicine consultations to people living with and beyond cancer with an emphasis on nutrition and cancer. He is also a general oncologist at Zuckerberg San Francisco General Hospital and Trauma Center.

Dr. Abrams was the president of the Society for Integrative Oncology in 2010 and has been a member of various education subcommittees of the American Society of Clinical Oncology. He was chief of the Hematology-Oncology Division at Zuckerberg San Francisco General from 2003-2017. He coedited the Oxford University Press textbook, *Integrative Oncology,* with Andrew Weil, MD. He was also named a "Top Cancer Doctor" in *Newsweek*'s 2015 Cancer issue, a special health issue exploring the challenges and innovations in cancer treatment and research.

Prior to specializing in oncology, Dr. Abrams worked in the field of HIV (Human Immunodeficiency Virus). He has served as assistant director of the UCSF Positive Health Program at San Francisco General Hospital and was chair of the Community Consortium, a professional association of more than 200 primary care providers treating Bay Area patients with HIV. He has conducted numerous clinical trials investigating complementary therapies in patients with HIV, including therapeutic touch, traditional Chinese medicine interventions, medical marijuana, medicinal mushrooms, and distant healing.

~ ~ ~

T. Colin Campbell, PhD, BS, MS, is the Jacob Gould Schurman Professor Emeritus of Nutritional Biochemistry at Cornell University, project director of the acclaimed China-Oxford-Cornell Diet and Health Project, coauthor of *The China Study*, and author of *Whole: Rethinking the Science of Nutrition.*

Dr. Campbell has been dedicated to the science of human health for more than 60 years. His primary focus is on the association between diet and disease, particularly cancer. Although largely known for *The China Study*—one of the most comprehensive studies of health and nutrition ever conducted and recognized by *The New York Times* as the "Grand Prix of epidemiology," Dr. Campbell's profound impact also includes extensive involvement in education, public policy, and laboratory research.

Dr. Campbell grew up on a dairy farm and studied at Cornell University (M.S., Ph.D.) and MIT (Research Associate) in nutrition, biochemistry and toxicology. He then spent 10 years on the faculty of Virginia Tech's Department of Biochemistry and Nutrition before returning to Cornell in 1975 where he presently holds his Endowed Chair as the Jacob Gould Schurman Professor Emeritus of Nutritional Biochemistry in the Division of Nutritional Sciences.

Dr. Campbell's research experience includes both laboratory experiments and large-scale human studies. He has received over 70 grant-years of peer-reviewed research funding (mostly with NIH), served on grant review panels of multiple funding agencies, actively participated in the development of national and international nutrition policy, and authored over 300 research papers. Throughout his career, he has confronted a great deal of confusion surrounding nutrition and its effects. In recent years, it is precisely this confusion that he has focused on so much

Dr. Campbell is also the author of *The New York Times* bestseller *Whole*, and *The Low-Carb Fraud*. He continues to share evidence-based information on health and nutrition whenever given the opportunity. He has delivered hundreds of lectures around the world and he is the founder of the T. Colin Campbell Center for Nutrition Studies and the online Plant-Based Nutrition Certificate in partnership with eCornell, an online learning company.

~ ~ ~

Alan Goldhamer, DC, is the founder of TrueNorth Health Center, a state-of-the-art facility that provides medical and chiropractic services, psychotherapy, and counseling.

Dr. Goldhamer is an outspoken professional who doesn't shy away from a spirited debate, he is deeply committed to helping people stuck in self-destructive cycles reclaim their ability to change their lives.

Dr. Goldhamer has supervised the water fasts of thousands of patients. Under his guidance, the Center has become one of the premier training facilities for doctors wishing to gain certification in the supervision of therapeutic fasting.

Dr. Goldhamer was the principal investigator in two landmark studies. The first: "Medically Supervised Water-Only Fasting in the Treatment of Hypertension" appeared in the June 2001 issue of the *Journal of Manipulative and Physiological Therapeutics*. Its publication marked a turning point in the evolution of evidence supporting the benefits of water-only fasting. The second study: "Medically Supervised Water-Only Fasting in the Treatment of Borderline Hypertension," appeared in the October 2002 issue of the *Journal of Alternative and Complementary Medicine*.

~ ~ ~

Michael Greger, MD FACLM, is a physician, New York Times bestselling author, and internationally recognized speaker on nutrition, food safety, and public health issues. A founding member and Fellow of the

American College of Lifestyle Medicine, Dr. Greger is licensed as a general practitioner specializing in clinical nutrition. He is a graduate of the Cornell University School of Agriculture and Tufts University School of Medicine. In 2017, Dr. Greger was honored with the ACLM Lifestyle Medicine Trailblazer Award and became a diplomat of the American Board of Lifestyle Medicine.

His latest books—*How Not to Die*, *The How Not to Die Cookbook*, and *How Not to Diet*—became instant New York Times Best Sellers. Dr. Greger has always donated to charity 100% of all proceeds he has ever received from his books, DVDs, and speaking engagements.

~ ~ ~

Michael Klaper, MD, is a gifted clinician, internationally recognized teacher, and sought-after speaker on diet and health. In addition to his clinical practice and private consultations with patients, he is a passionate and devoted educator of physicians and other healthcare professionals about the importance of nutrition in clinical practice and integrative medicine.

Dr. Klaper graduated from the University of Illinois College of Medicine in 1972 and is currently a member of the American College of Lifestyle Medicine as well as serving on the Advisory Board for the Plantrician Project™ and the *International Journal of Disease Reversal and Prevention.*

Dr. Klaper, in conjunction with the non-profit PlantPure Communities (PPC), has launched the Moving Medicine Forward initiative with the goal to engage a growing group of new supporters to help kindle the flame of nutritional-awareness in the minds of medical students across North America and to have applied nutrition routinely taught at every medical school.

~ ~ ~

Gordon Saxe, MD, PhD., MPH, is the Director of the UC San Diego Center for Integrative Nutrition and Chair of the Krupp Endowment for research on the benefits of natural complementary and alternative medicine; he is a preventive and integrative medicine physician, and co-developer of the UCSD Natural Healing & Cooking Program. He is also the recipient of a prestigious NIH Career Development Award from the National Center for Complementary and Alternative Medicine.

Dr. Saxe is a national expert in cancer and complementary and alternative medicine and is most well-known for his pioneering work in the combined use of a plant-based diet and body-mind stress reduction to control the progression of advanced prostate cancer. His previous studies have included: epidemiology of diet and cancers of prostate, breast, and pancreas; diet and body-mind exercise to control the spread of advanced prostate cancer; and diet and gene expression in prostate cancer. He received his MD at Michigan State University, his PhD in Epidemiology at the University of Michigan, and his MPH in Nutrition at Tulane University.

~ ~ ~

Although I did not have a chance to do an interview with **Dr. John McDougall,** he provided me a treasure trove of solid research data related to prostate cancer and its treatment. I also was very liberal in using his web resources and his personal summaries and analyses he provides on his website. Dr. McDougall is a physician and nutrition expert who teaches better health through vegetarian cuisine. He has been studying, writing, and speaking out about the effects of nutrition on disease for over 50 years. He is the founder and director of the nationally renowned McDougall Program, a ten-day residential program that he and his wife Mary McDougall host at a luxury resort in Santa Rosa, CA, where medical miracles occur through diet and lifestyle change. His program not only promotes a broad range of dramatic and lasting health benefits but, most importantly, can also reverse serious illnesses including high blood pressure, heart disease, diabetes, and others—all without the use of drugs.

A graduate of Michigan State University's College of Human Medicine, Dr. McDougall performed his internship at Queen's Medical Center in Honolulu, Hawaii, and his medical residency at the University of Hawaii. He and Mary are also the authors of several nationally best-selling books, including their most recent, *The Starch Solution*.

~ ~ ~

My wife, Mindy, will also add her personal perspectives to this book, coming from her heart as she shares with us the caregiver's viewpoint. As you have probably discovered, your support team plays a crucial role in your health and healing. The caregiver's journey can be just as difficult as ours (we who are afflicted), and possibly sometimes harder if the caregivers are our spouses or loved ones.

~ ~ ~

You might not have even pulled the most powerful card out of your hand yet in your cancer battle. This is a book of inspiration and hope. You have more power over your outcome than you know.

PART 1

CHAPTER 1
WHO AM I?

Life's biggest tragedy is that we get old too soon and wise too late.

— Benjamin Franklin

I feel like I have lived in two boxes in my life. The first box was the "I'm going-to-live-forever box." In this box, life is glorious. I had a great career, an awesome (and very hot) wife, three great kids, a high-paying job with a flexible schedule that allowed me time to surf more days a week than not. I love to surf. In the "I'm going-to-live-forever box," the food and liquor are unlimited. I was consistently eating well over 3000 calories a day of disease-promoting food, consuming at least two martinis each evening, and I thought that was just fine. When I DID go to the doctor, I noticed that my blood pressure and cholesterol were going up throughout my 30s and 40s. No problem. I, like many Americans, assumed that this was not serious, just a few biomarkers that I would address at some point in the future, but not today. Life seemed pretty good in the "I am going-to-live-forever box."

Life wasn't good because I was in complete denial and fooling myself. I was firmly implanted in my "I am going-to-live-forever box" which was also my "I'm not gonna die" box. My weight went from 155 (college weight) to 177 pounds by the time I was 47. My cholesterol, which had always been too high, had now reached the dangerous level of 276. I had convinced myself that letting the notches out of my belt to accommodate an increasingly large gut was just, well, normal and part of aging. I was spending at least 2-3 nights out with business associates, which is more or less code for "let's eat really rich food and get lit with liquor" and call it customer relations! My doctor never said one single word about nutrition or diet. Changing my diet didn't even cross my mind in my 30s and 40s.

At age 53, I read a book—just by accident really, called *The China Study* by Dr. T. Colin Campbell. Mindy and I were flying across the country, and I forgot my trashy novel which I was reading; so out of sheer boredom, I started reading Mindy's book. Little did I know that what I was reading would change the trajectory of the rest of my life. What I read had me floored. Why didn't I know this information? I knew nothing about the relationship food has to do with our health. Why wasn't this common knowledge? I went from carnivore to herbivore on that six-hour plane flight and dropped my cholesterol by over 100 points over the next six weeks. When I met with my doc to brag about what I had done all he had to say was, "Your PSA is high."

Chapter 1 – Who Am I?

I stepped into the "Holy shit, I'm-gonna-die box" the day I got the call from my urologist letting me know I had PC.

Mindy (my one-and-only wife of close to 40 years) and I currently live in a 32-foot 2008 Winnebago Sunrise RV. Our RV, aka "The Wellness Wagon," is a mobile billboard. You can't miss us traveling down the road. The RV is wrapped in fruits and vegetables with our non-profit logo, "One Day to Wellness," emblazoned on all sides. It's ridiculous and over the top. Just what we wanted.

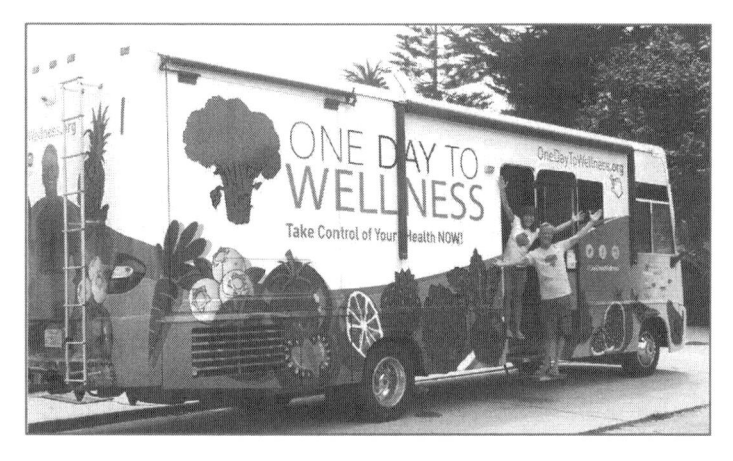

We are traveling nomads and lecture all over the world on nutrition and fitness. We chose this life because we know there is currently nothing more important than helping people understand the relationship between the foods we eat (or don't eat) and our health and happiness outcomes. I am fully committed here, with a very strong

PURPOSE. My experience has taught me that having a purpose is critical to cancer survival and a life well lived.

Summary

1. Don't wait for a chronic disease diagnosis to change your behavior. A health crisis like PC takes decades to develop into a life-threatening disease.
2. Acknowledge NOW that what you eat every day is the powerful impact on your long-term health.
3. Make sure you have a purpose and let that focus fuel your heart and health.

CHAPTER 2
WHY DON'T WE KNOW

It's possible to be so ignorant that you do not know how ignorant you are.

Anonymous

The leading cause of death and disability in the United States is the food we place in our mouths each day, according to "The Global Burden of Disease Study," funded by the Bill and Melinda Gates Foundation. This massive study looked at dietary consumption between 1990 and 2017 in 195 countries, focusing on 15 types of food or nutrients. Investigators concluded that, due to its contribution to non-communicable diseases, poor diet accounted for 1 in 5, or 11 million, adult deaths in 2017.[1]

Most of us (me included) have learned to rely on our doctors to be the best source of the latest nutritional information, yet it turns out our physicians get less than 20 hours of nutritional education in medical school![2]

And this might surprise you: Only 27% of medical schools even HAVE a course on nutrition.[3]

That's why, unless your personal physician has made the effort to educate him or herself on evidence-based nutrition, at their own expense, after medical school, with no hope of reimbursement, they probably are not aware of this vital life-saving information covered in the pages to follow. It's not their fault.

Having spent a lot of time and money with the best urologists, oncologists, and radiologists in the country, the subject of nutrition was brought up very rarely or not at all. When I broached the subject during a doctors' meeting, the idea of nutrition having an impact on anyone's treatment outcome was shrugged off or considered misguided patient mumbo jumbo.

There have been a few exceptions to this, and thankfully, I have been fortunate enough to have built what I consider to be a strong team of oncological specialists with Prostate Oncology Specialists (PROS) in Marina Del Rey, CA, coupled with one of the best local oncologists here in Santa Cruz, CA, where we live. (We actually travel full time, but we do have a home!) Up until connecting with Dr. Scholz, Dr. Turner, and their team at PROS, diet was not on the menu of items to discuss. Diet is key and more on this later, but even with the best of the best, I have learned that I am the boss, and I am skippering my own ship with nutrition and lifestyle modifications. I have control over these things, and as I mentioned, lifestyle and diet are the very things that probably got me here in the first place. Remember, you are the boss, and you need the best support team you can find. But even the best of the best, in all likelihood, had little or no formally taught nutritional classes during their time in medical school. The best medical doctors can deliver the best medical treatment, but usually, they aren't prepared for or are capable of discussing and delivering the vital nutritional and emotional treatment we all need after diagnosis. I have learned you have to do that yourself. For the first time in my life, I have taken control of my own health, and it is the most empowering thing I have ever done. You can too!

I have a unique perspective. I have spent the last nine years of my life battling prostate cancer, which is not unusual. However, I have spent about the same amount of time studying evidence-based nutritional science, becoming an advocate and public speaker on how whole-food plant-based nutrition changed my life for the better and continues to do so today. As my knowledge and application of nutrition as a critical adjunct treatment in my cancer care regimen grew and helped me deal with treatment/recovery/treatment/recovery, I became shocked at how supposedly the most advanced cancer care system in the world (ours), still to this day, even with the mountain of scientific evidence to support it, almost completely ignores nutrition as an integral treatment regime, adjunct, or otherwise. I have news for you: NUTRITION IS IMPORTANT! Really, really, important. Probably THE most important issue that contributes to PC development, and also, I believe, the most important issue to address after receiving your diagnosis.

According to an article published in the *Journal of the National Cancer,* researchers found that of the 53 cancer drugs that were approved during the period 2003–2013 by the FDA and the European Medicines Agency (EMA), only 43% improved overall survival by three or more months and 45% were associated with reduced safety. Sixteen (30%) of the approved drugs failed to demonstrate any improvement in overall survival. Indeed, many recently introduced drugs fail to meet the benchmark of producing the clinically meaningful outcomes promoted by the American Society of Clinical Oncology (ASCO) Cancer Research Committee. [4]

This is why I had to write this book. There is a vital missing link in our cancer care specifically and in our health care system at large:

> Acknowledgement that nutrition plays a critical role in both the development of cancer as well as its treatment and recovery.

My hope is to help men just like me begin to develop and then cultivate this understanding. That's basically all the men who are or will be dealing with prostate cancer, and there are over two million of us walking around right now. We are all going to take our own medical approach to this devastating diagnosis, but ignoring nutritional approaches to prostate cancer is dangerous. I follow the science. The science is very, very good. So good, it forced me to change my behavior and as a result, my life.

Chapter 2 – Why Don't We Know

The truth is that nine years have passed since my diagnosis, and having endured all the standard treatments and knowing the cancer is still there and growing, I feel better mentally, physically, and emotionally than I ever have in my life. I attribute most of this to my change in diet. How bizarre. But not really. As my knowledge and understanding of the undeniably strong relationship between diet and PC grew, and as I met with more and more doctors and medical professionals who treat cancer, I became increasingly frustrated that the cancer medical community in particular (because I am living in it) has not embraced the power of diet in prostate cancer treatment. It stuns me, and I want to do something about it.

~ ~ ~

Expert analysis—Dr. T Colin Campbell

This goes back to a question that I came to understand from the 1800s. There were two ideas of what cancer is: local or constitutional. That was a prominent debate in the 1800s.

If it's a local disease which the surgeons like to advocate, that means it's localized, and we'll cut it out. So it's simple. The alternative hypothesis was that cancer is a reflection of something larger going on with our bodies, which would tend to encompass environment, food, and so forth.

So we had these two views and some reasonable debates on this through the 1800s. And then the local theory sort of won out. The surgeons were powerful, and they had their way.

Then the debate then came about for breast cancer. Now the surgeons were joined by people who wanted to solve this local disease by zapping it with a narrow beam of radiation in late 1890s.

Then people had the idea of—why don't we find a chemical that can zap that target? One of the first attempts was being given to breast cancer patients. Ridiculous, but they were advocating that at the time. And so the whole idea was finding some chemical that could do that. The idea was that those chemicals would work best if they were very selective. The idea was to kill the cancer cells with chemicals that obviously were toxic. They called them cytotoxic chemotherapy, and the chemicals could maybe zap the cancer and not cause the side effects because no drugs can do that.

That's the power of the whole as I described it in my book, *Whole (Whole: Rethinking the Science of Nutrition)*.

Chapter 2 – Why Don't We Know

The complete body is working together. How can you go through a haystack and find that needle without poking, you know, something like that?

The doctors have such a difficult time with something like this. Of course, they are not trained in the first sense, but in the even worse sense, they are not trained on the concept of whole-ism because they have been trained in reductionism. So, they're still looking for the local effect. They're still looking for this single thing that's going to zap something, kill something, so forth, and so on.

We need to back off from that idea. Look at not only prostate cancer but other cancers and heart disease and all the rest. It's the same solution across the board, essentially, for all this sort of stuff. And it turns out, it's just eating plants. You know, not eating animals. I mean, I never thought I'd say that when I was younger, but, you know, not eating animals, eating plants. And then not making use of some of the products of the modern day like extracts, you know, like a vitamin pulled out of a plant, or like fat being pulled out of plants like corn oil, cooking oils.

Summary

1. Nutrition has a vitally important role to play in the development and also the progression of PC.
2. Even today, doctors receive very little education on nutrition.
3. Don't wait for the medical system to catch up with science. Implement WFPB (Whole-Food, Plant-Based) nutrition now.

CHAPTER 3
THE DAY THAT CHANGED MY LIFE

Stop looking for health where you lost it.

— Anonymous

December 11th, 2011, is the day that changed my life forever and the lives of the people most important to me. Chances are you had a very similar experience if you bought this book. This may have been my first mistake that you can learn from. SLOW DOWN. I was in my kitchen in Santa Cruz with my wife, Mindy, when my urologist called. As soon as I picked up the phone, I knew it was bad news.

"Yes, Bruce, your biopsy came back two positive cores out of eight—you have prostate cancer."

My knees went wobbly, vision blurred, complete confusion, no, no, no. NO……Yes. Oh, God. I want it OUT! NOW!……………………………….

From then on, time began to blur with anxiety and fear. I did not feel connected to reality. Beyond being stunned, crushed, unable to link thoughts, I remember telling my urologist that I wanted to come in immediately to discuss options and arranged for an appointment that same afternoon. At the most important time in my life to have a sharp mind, slow down, and make deliberate, thought-out decisions, my mind had transitioned to a state of fight-or-flight stress response that completely debilitated my decision-making capability for the foreseeable future. The foreseeable future is when I would have to make decisions that were going to change my life forever. This was NOT a good formula or frame of mind for making smart choices about prostate cancer treatment.

But this is what we all are confronted with on the day when we get THAT call.

~ ~ ~

Mindy's Perspective

In 27 years of marriage, I had never seen my husband falter in any way. He was our rock in our crazy sea of raising three boys, all hell-bent to break mom in one way or another. Don't get me wrong, our boys are and have always been the light of our lives, but three very active boys and a mom who feeds off that energy requires a dedicated, even-keeled dad present. That's what Bruce always was—steady and reliable in a very even-keeled sort of way. He was always prepared to deflect emotional disturbance. I later learned that this was a coping mechanism Bruce set up for himself to navigate an emotionally turbulent childhood.

When that cancer diagnosis call came, the man I had known for 27 years collapsed in one split second into emotional mush. I was ill-prepared for this and had no tools in my toolbox to help in any way. I wanted to fix him. I needed to make it all better—NOW. What do I say? What do I do? I started saying whatever I could think of. "It will all be alright." "We will get through this." Blah Blah Blah. Words and more words. What Bruce needed at that moment, I would later realize, was just to know that I was close. Not to say anything. Not to try to make it better. Just to be there.

Through the ups and downs, I have learned that less is better. And that I can't fix IT. I am here, and that is enough.

Summary

1. Do not make decisions based on fear. You have more time than you think to sort through this initial shock.
2. Push fear aside and take your time to learn ALL of your options, not just what your doctor or oncologist is suggesting. This is not the time for fast decision making.
3. From the caregiver's perspective—sometimes less is more. The caregiver's job is not to fix but to listen and support.

CHAPTER 4
HOW DID I GET HERE?

Ignorance is not bliss—it is oblivion.

— Philip Wylie

Early Years

I was born in Atlanta, GA, on May 18th, 1958, in the heart of the baby boom and was very fortunate to have grown up when and where I did. I had loving parents who cared for all my needs. Bottle feeding was in, and so I was a bottle-fed baby along with being fed all the processed baby food products that were just coming onto the market. I remember that the first field trip I took was in the first grade, and we went to—of course—the Coca-Cola Headquarters. New types of food-like products were appearing faster than the old ones were disappearing. In the sixties, our country's progress and prosperity in space and technology emboldened the food industry. If we could land someone on the moon, we could certainly do a better job of creating food than nature does. And we tried, and the food-like products were tasty, and I was on the eager end of reception. I always loved food of all kinds.

In Atlanta, GA, fried Chicken is a food group, and Coca-Cola is considered a sacred institution. I often look back now when I was growing up. I have wonderful memories of family and friends, but when I think of what I ate, I pretty much come up with the following menu or a derivative of it.

Breakfast:
- Pop-tarts were my staple.
- Lots of instant Carnation powdered milk things.
- Eggs prepared every way imaginable.
- Sausage and or bacon at almost every breakfast when there was time.
- Whole milk. At least one glass with every meal, milkshakes, yogurt, cheese, and cheese.
- Processed packaged sugary cereal—Captain Crunch was my personal favorite.

Snack:
- Milkshake with a raw egg! Yum!

Lunch:
- Almost always a luncheon meat on white bread with mayo.
- Chips almost every day—hell, every day for 54 years. (Side note—I am a recovering chip-aholic. If there are free potato chips in the hotel lobby bar, I have to find another hotel to stay at.)
- Cookies and pastries and candy, candy, candy.

Dinner:
- TV dinners (lots and lots).
- My mom usually made dinner, but it was always meat-centered.
- Dark leafy green vegetables were simply unheard of. Vegetables at our house usually came out of a can or a frozen plastic bag which probably explains why I never cared for them.
- Ice cream and pie or cake for dessert every night.

That was the SAD (Standard American Diet) of my youth. As an adult, I augmented my SAD diet with excessive alcohol consumption in my mid-20s that lasted into my 50s right up to my PC diagnosis—the alcohol stayed part of my diet for longer because I had convinced myself that alcohol was plant-based. This, I believe, is the core culprit of me developing cancer. After absorbing all the research on PC and lifestyle, I just can't come up with any other logical conclusion. There are no absolutes and no guarantees, but there are a lot of "smoking guns" in my cancer development, and I think it's important to acknowledge them so I could start climbing out of the grave I was digging with my teeth for most of my life.

With the knowledge we now have about the eating patterns of countries that have higher (and I mean much higher) rates of PC compared to the rest of the world, I have come to the conclusion that I kept fueling prostate cancer for decades without realizing it. According to the

International Agency for Cancer Research (IACR), the US is ranked #2 in PC cases, with Australia in the #1 spot.[1] Who are the top two meat and dairy consuming countries of the world? The USA and Australia.[2] The Western eating patterns of low nutrient, high fat, high cholesterol, and animal-based foods are directly associated with increasing rates of prostate cancer worldwide.[3]

According to the World Cancer Research Fund, prostate cancer is the second most commonly occurring cancer in men and the fourth most commonly occurring cancer overall. There were 1.3 million new cases in 2018.[4]

My diet for my whole life was pretty much junk food, fried animal products, and excessive dairy in the form of, well, everything. And I was a skinny kid. I could eat anything I wanted, and it never caused me problems, and I never gained weight (until my 30s and 40s, and uh......50s).

Was nutrition ever discussed at the dinner table at my house? Never. That was the way it was with almost everybody, and unfortunately, this tradition still holds true for most families today. We continue to overlook food and the relationship it has to our health. Isn't the saying, "You are what you eat" true? Yes, it is, but up until recently, we simply did not know all the details. But now we do, and all we have to do is open our eyes and see the data.

World Health Organization Prostate Cancer Incidence and Mortality Rates Globally

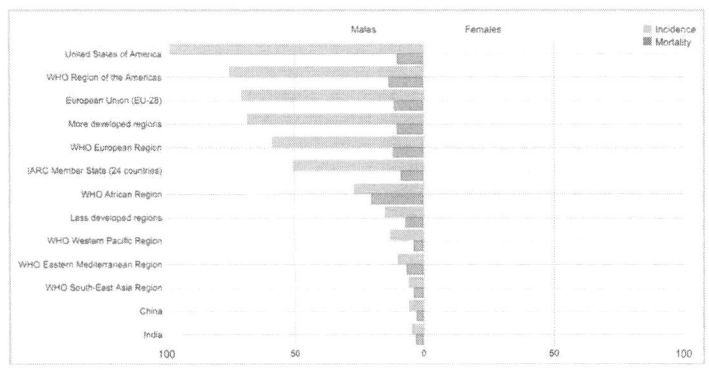

	Incidence	Mortality
United States of America		
WHO Region of the Americas		
European Union (EU-28)		
More developed regions		
WHO European Region		
IARC Member Stats (24 countries)		
WHO African Region		
Less developed regions		
WHO Western Pacific Region		
WHO Eastern Mediterranean Region		
WHO South-East Asia Region		
China		
India		

These numbers are x 1000

If you are going to eat the Standard American Diet (SAD) like I did for 53 years, your odds of developing prostate cancer are MUCH higher than average. Genes do play a role, but as I learned from Dr. Campbell, they never act alone. I had to have the right genetic make-up to develop cancer, but one thing is certain: I promoted the growth and expansion of the cancer in my body with a poor diet for many decades.

Middle Years

When I was 13, my family moved from Atlanta, GA, to Orlando, FL. My dad was tiring of corporate management life and planned on taking advantage of the explosive growth the Walt Disney Company was fueling in the greater Orlando area as a developer. Life was great as a teenager living on a lake in Central Florida. We had a ski boat which is where I spent most of my time. My high school years were filled with—let's just say I came of age in the 70s. What do you think I did? PARTY! I did not avoid the temptations of the privileged high-school student, experimenting with alcohol and cannabis, just like all of my friends.

I don't "party" like I did in high school or college, but I still eat every day. And as I look back and compare what I ate most of my life to how I eat now, the juxtaposition is stark and drastic. When I look back and try to fill in my mental food log during my high school years, I come up with pretty much the same diet I ate as a child:

Breakfast:
- Usually, none or pop-tarts or Captain Crunch cereal or a two or three-egg omelet.

Lunch:
- Giant turkey or roast beef sandwich at the deli every day. No exception. Always with chips and a Coca Cola.

Snacks:
- Candy bars

Dinner:
- Top-ramen
- Fast food
- Lots of southern barbeque
- All dinners were always finished with ice-cream

I could have cared less about nutrition in high school. But looking back now through the lens of someone who is focused on consuming health-promoting foods, I just don't recall eating anything healthful and certainly not on PURPOSE.

College was much the same and probably even worse as I was never home for a home-cooked meal. Mostly, it was four years of eating ramen topped with an egg. I went to the University of Florida and graduated in June of 1980. I ended up getting a BA in Economics, which turned out to be a great educational base for the rest of my life. I grabbed the diploma, got in my car, and drove to California without a second thought. As I mentioned, we lived on a lake with a ski boat in Florida. My friends and I loved to ski, but we began experimenting with surfing behind the wake of the ski-boat and I was bitten by the surfing bug. This is important, because from age 13 on, surfing has played a pivotal and instrumental role in my life and in dealing with cancer. I was hooked on surfing and still am to this day. That's why I ended up in Santa Cruz, CA.

Summary

1. The modern western diet is strongly associated with an increased risk of developing PC.
2. Moving away from the SAD diet to a WFPB diet will have a positive impact on your health at any age.
3. The decisions you make in your 20s, 30s, and 40s matter.

CHAPTER 5
TURNING POINTS

Warren Buffett may know more about smart investing than any other human on the planet, but he outdid himself when he openly shared what he calls the biggest decision of his life: marriage. Well, not just marriage, but picking the right person to marry. As the billionaire told his shareholders at a 2009 Berkshire annual meeting: "Marry the right person. I'm serious about that. It will make more difference in your life. It will change your aspirations, all kinds of things."

— Business Insider

For the first six months after I graduated from college, I worked part-time in the evenings at what was at the time Long's Drug Store in downtown Santa Cruz, so I could surf during daylight hours every day. My core food group: Fast Mexican Food—It's everywhere in California, and it's delicious! After surfing myself silly for six months, I realized I needed to establish a more serious long-term career plan other than surfing and stocking shelves in a drug store. I was in the right place at the right time. I got a job in purchasing at a high-tech startup in Silicon Valley, which jumpstarted my career in sales and marketing. I quickly transitioned into an account rep position in the semiconductor industry and never looked back.

The first major turning point in my adult life happened in 1980, when I met my wife, Mindy. This was the single biggest and best thing that has ever happened to me. Period. We fell in love immediately.

We got married in 1983 and moved from our condo in San Jose to Santa Cruz. I commuted to my job in "The Valley" where business was booming. For the next 25 years, I lived the Silicon Valley fast-paced lifestyle, raised a family of three boys with Mindy, and surfed. It was awesome. For most of my sales career, I had a company credit card which, although not specifically stated, was earmarked for customer entertainment. The goal of every company I worked for was to spend as much "off the clock" time with clients as possible. What better way to do that than to buy them lunch, dinner, and drinks? And that is what I did almost every day.

I was a master at ignoring the clear signs of my declining health. My blood pressure steadily climbed along with my cholesterol and weight. I told myself that that was just the way it was like so many people I know. The key that unlocked the bullshit door on me was the

Chapter 5 – Turning Points

meeting I had with my family physician when I was 46. This was to be the second biggest turning point in my adult life. My appointment with the doctor went something like this, "Bruce, your cholesterol is climbing, and you are at risk of a cardiovascular event. In addition, you have high blood pressure, and your triglycerides are elevated. I noticed on your chart that your father has heart disease and that your grandfather also died of a heart attack in his early 70s. Because of your family history of heart disease, I think it would be wise to put you on a course of statin drugs to bring down your cholesterol. This is VERY common. After that, we need to look at possible beta-blockers for your high blood pressure."

This was not what I was expecting. My annual visit to the doctor was primarily to score sleeping pills because I was spending so much time flying back and forth across the country. At that time in my career, I was the west coast sales manager for a company based out of Boston, so at least twice a month, I was flying across the country swapping time zones. I didn't go into the doc's office for a lecture on my health, I went in for sleeping pills. Now here I am with this dude telling me I need to go on drugs for the rest of my life to prevent myself from dying of a heart attack! Really? I was still in denial at this point, I was comfortable in my "I am-going-to-live-forever box," eating and drinking whatever I wanted, not sleeping enough, and at the height of my family financial responsibility curve.

I woke up the next morning, shook off my usual hangover, and drove the hour to my office from Santa

Cruz to San Jose (minimum one-hour drive to the office every day on top of all of the other bad habits I had accumulated and nurtured over a lifetime). That one hour got me thinking—really thinking. Thinking about making some changes in my life.

I parked, went into my office, and shut the door and called Mindy. She had been persistently nudging me to go into business with her in the fitness world for the last decade. Her career was on FIRE, and she was doing exactly what she wanted to do. She had become THE most popular fitness instructor in Silicon Valley, competed and won both the National and World Aerobic Championships (Aerobics and group exercise were huge in the 80s and 90s), teaching at every fitness conference, and, now she just landed her first infomercial host gig with what turned out to be a huge success. The "Six Second Abs" infomercial turned out to be my escape ticket from corporate America. Up to this point, I had never seriously considered the leap into another career primarily because we had a mortgage and three kids headed to college. And up to this point, Mindy's income was meager. But that meeting with the doctor had affected me. Was I living my best life now? Mindy had wanted us to join forces and go into business together for years, and now seemed like the right time.

When the first royalty check came in, I suddenly became THE biggest fan of "Six Second Abs!" This was serious money! Suddenly (for some reason the decision came about 45 seconds after that first royalty check arrived in the mail), I realized that the corporate world was not for me anymore. In truth, I had an awesome experience working in "The Valley." Right place, right time. I loved the pace, I loved sales, I loved the money, but the start-up I was working was becoming non-start-upish and more corporate. I was also burned-out, which is a common chronic condition for just about everyone working in high-tech. And that first royalty check of Mindy's ......wow.

Summary

1. Find a great lifelong partner.
2. Don't ignore the early signs of chronic disease (ED, high blood pressure, etc.).
3. Take more risk than you are comfortable with.

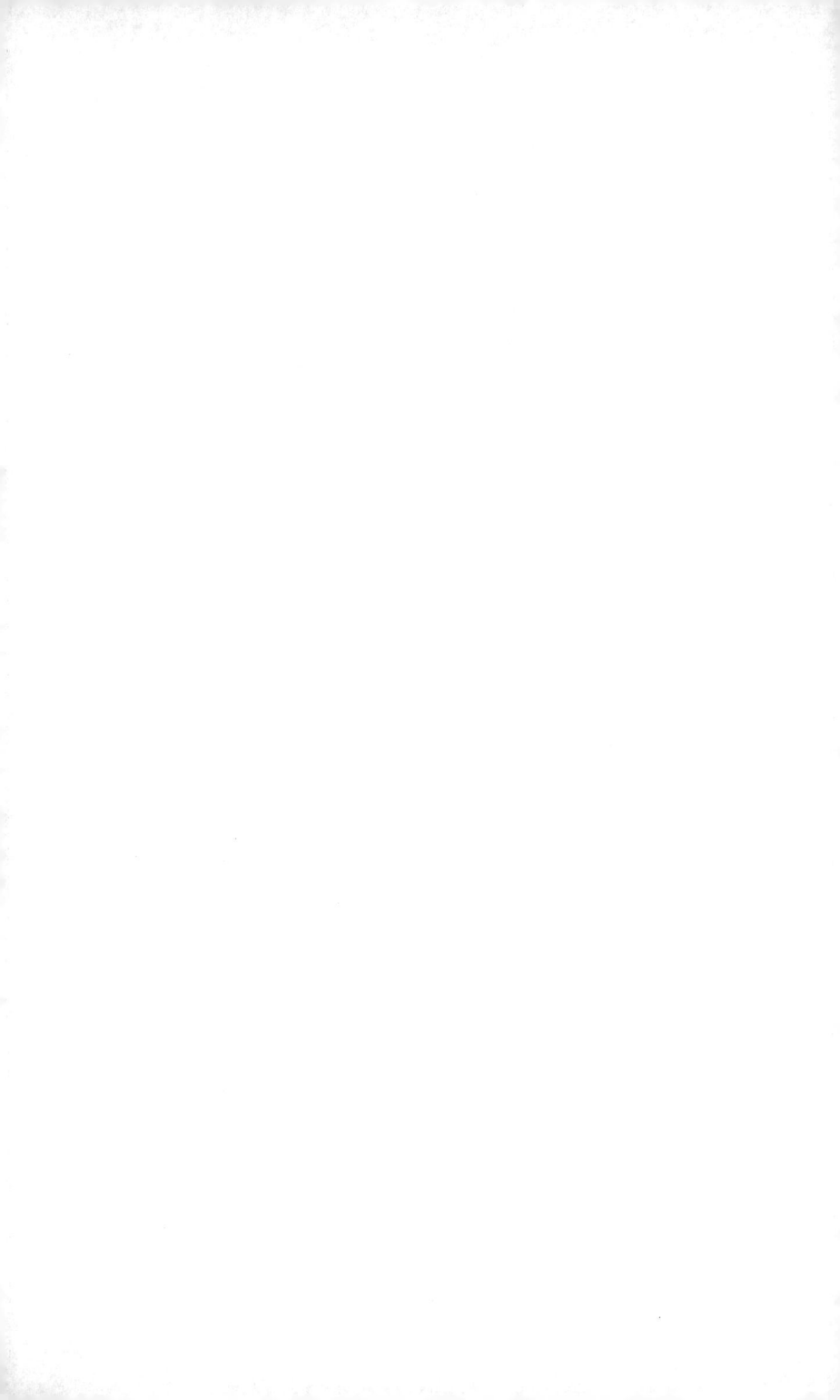

CHAPTER 6
WORKING FOR MYSELF

Once you decide to work for yourself, you never go back to work for somebody else.

— Alan Sugar

Mindy and I agreed that we would put together a business plan for our new fledgling company. That was it. Decision made. I called my boss the next day, and after 12 years of employment with this company, I asked him to lay me off so I could get a severance package which he did, but not without first counseling me on the perils of going it alone—and more so—about the dangers of going into business with your wife.

I got almost one year of severance! I remember mapping out on our wall calendar with a red magic marker how long I would receive severance before it stopped. I figured after a year we would know if we could make it or not.

I left the corporate world and never looked back. Mindy and I were, and still are, in business together.

Mindy was the talent, and I began marketing and selling the products and exercise programs she had developed with the infomercial company. We also launched at the same time, a fitness video production company (FitFlix Productions), and a series of fitness conferences around the country (FitFest). We theorized that if we launched a few programs and products, at least one would come to fruition. I knew nothing about the fitness industry, but with Mindy's passion, popularity, and knowledge, within a year, we had a thriving fitness video production company, a great series of national events, and had begun selling Mindy's latest blockbuster product—the Gliding Discs. Gliding discs are now a standard piece of exercise equipment in every gym in the world. Go, Mindy!

We were working nonstop, traveling nonstop, and pushing ourselves to the max. It was awesome!

But back to my health. As I mentioned, at the peak of my body bloating when I had that fateful meeting with my doctor in 2002, I weighed about 176 pounds (I am 5' 10"). This may not seem like a lot, especially now with the world being overweight, but I had the big paunch and a full puffy face that comes along with being FAT.

As soon as I left the corporate world, I started losing weight. I wasn't commuting two-plus hours a day, and I could surf whenever I wanted. I worked out with Mindy regularly, and I was beginning to dabble in shopping and cooking for the family. This meant no more expense account to take out clients and eat and drink whatever I wanted. I was beginning to lose weight, but unfortunately, it was not soon enough. I had no idea yet, but PC had taken hold inside my body and was on the move.

Summary

1. Commit to your dream but have a plan and a back-up plan.
2. Having a financial buffer is crucial to stress management.
3. Going into business with your spouse is awesome—unless it isn't. Make sure you have a relationship that will withstand both roles of business and life partner

CHAPTER 7
FINDING NUTRITIONAL RESEARCH AND DISCOVERING THE TRUTH

There'll always be serendipity involved in discovery.

— Jeff Bezos

This was the third pivotal turning point in my life. Mindy and I were flying across the country in 2011. Our business was running on all cylinders, and so were we. We flew somewhere almost every week to a conference or training. This particular trip took us from San Francisco to Myrtle Beach, South Carolina, for yet another conference. Our good friend, Jessica Maurer, had given Mindy the book, *The China Study,* by T. Colin Campbell for her 50th birthday (thank you, Jessica), and Mindy brought it on the plane with her. I was bored, saw the book, and started reading. My life has never been the same (thank you, Dr. Campbell). I read almost the entire book in four hours.

I am a data-driven person. If you work in high tech in Silicon Valley, you have no choice but to become data and science driven, or at least literate. I don't know how else to put it, but I was completely stunned by what I read in this book. Dr. Campbell's approach was all elegantly data driven and came to a very solid conclusion about the problem with our diet in this country and its tight link to ALL chronic diseases, not just prostate cancer. (Reminder: I still did not know I had cancer on this flight in the spring of 2011.) In behavioral-change terminology, I am a diver.

When I study something and mentally approve the sources and their subsequent suggestions, I do my best to go all in. And so it went on this flight across the country. I am not going to dive into the details of *The China Study* here, but please go buy the book and read it if you haven't. Dr. Campbell's conclusions are echoed in the interview I had with him about his career, nutrition, and prostate cancer.

I got on the plane—a sanctimonious, heavy, meat-eating, standard American kind of guy. The book kicked my ass back down to admitting I had basically a nursery school understanding of what good nutrition is. I went from completely humbled to really pissed off on that four-plus hour plane ride. I just could not believe that I had not heard this information before. I was (or so I thought) a really intelligent sales and marketing exec in one of the most technologically advanced industries on the planet. I was being paid good money! I was an idiot.

Two weeks prior to this enlightenment, and I can think of no better word, I was again sitting in my doc's

Chapter 7 – Finding Nutritional Research and...

office being told I needed to go on statins for the rest of my life to control my cholesterol and not keel over in my 50s of a heart attack. No mention of dietary intervention. EVER. And now I have just finished reading a groundbreaking book by one of the most respected nutritional scientists in the world with the basic message that:

> Most cancers, including prostate cancer, as well as heart disease and diabetes, are preventable and directly related to life-long eating patterns. In addition, changing eating behavior and removing the foods that we know cause these conditions can, in many cases, reverse the disease process and bring the body back to a healthy state—without drugs, without surgery, without supplements, and without spending hundreds of thousands of dollars.

There it was—with extensive population, epidemiological, lab, and clinical studies to back up the claim. Dr. Campbell also specifically stated with tremendous proof that you could bring down high cholesterol levels to very healthy levels simply by transitioning to eating a plant-based diet. WHAT? I had never read or heard of such a thoroughly researched book on the science of nutrition. Surely every doctor knows about this, right? Why on earth did my doctor not mention any of this to me? Was he just an ill-informed bad doctor? He knows I don't want to take statins. I was furious. This is where I learned a shocking and embarrassing truth about the medical profession:

> How we eat is the primary driver of 80% to 90% of the chronic health conditions we suffer and die from in this country. And as I mentioned earlier, medical students STILL get little or no education in nutrition or nutritional counseling. My doctor was not a bad doctor; he simply was completely ignorant about the field of nutrition. And like so many doctors, he had learned that the way to manage chronic conditions, like high cholesterol, was, of course, with DRUGS! Which would be awesome and easy. The only problem is that every single major drug that has been developed to treat high blood pressure, high cholesterol, diabetes/pre-diabetes, and I'll even put Lupron for treating PC in this category as well, are designed and targeted to treat the symptoms of the specific bio-marker, not the root cause of the problem itself.

So here I am standing outside the baggage claim at the Myrtle Beach Airport for a three-day conference, and I am a different person. After 52 years of eating a meat, dairy, junk-food SAD diet (I am still in recovery as a French fry and potato chip addict), I had just learned vital life-saving information from a very credible team of scientists with Dr. Campbell leading the way. As I stood there, I confronted myself with the most daunting challenge of my life. (PC takes the prize for most daunting, but I was still blissfully unaware I even had the disease.) I was compelled to change. I did not want to suffer from heart disease as I watched my father do for most of his adult life. And I now realized that I could achieve that. I made a commitment to myself that day that I would become a whole-food plant-based eater at least long enough to determine if I could bring my cholesterol down to a safe level.

Summary

1. Start using the incredible resources available to you listed in the back of this book.
2. Let science and research lead your decision making—not ego, outdated beliefs, or lifelong food preferences and addictions.
3. It is never too late to learn something new and to turn that knowledge into action.

CHAPTER 8
THIS IS THE DEFINITION OF A TURNING POINT—EAT THE FOOD!

You don't have to see the whole staircase. Just take the first step.

— Martin Luther King, Jr.

One book, one plane flight, and I was now a vegan in my brain. But I hadn't actually changed my behavior and ATE THE FOOD. *So what does a newly empowered vegan do?* I mused. I could go out to the beautifully manicured lawn in front of the airport and begin grazing on the grass. This situation for me was analogous to a new architect showing up for work and very excited, except the only knowledge of architecture he or she has is from thumbing through *Architectural Digest.* What am I supposed to do now? Whole Foods! I remembered seeing some of my now fellow vegans going into that store and eating at… the…. salad bar. Just salad.

A new Whole Foods had just opened up just north of Myrtle Beach. Our original plan was to head straight to a barbecue joint, as South Carolina touts itself as being the barbecue capital of the USA. Change of plans.

I quickly informed Mindy that I was now a vegan and that we were going to go to Whole Foods for dinner, not barbecue. She looked at me like I was from another planet. Prior to this trip, I had been internet trolling the best barbecue joints in the area, and I was verbally excited about sucking down some of the best baby back spare ribs in the world. Mindy does not like barbecue and was more than happy to go to Whole Foods.

As we pulled into the parking lot, this new vegan was now anxious and fearful. I was familiar with the WF (Whole Foods) salad bar as I had walked past it dozens of times on my way to the incredible cheese, dairy, and meat sections of the store. To the salad bar I marched!! I proudly built myself a complete plant-based salad meal just like a good vegan would do. One problem: As you probably know, directly next and parallel to the salad bar at WF is the hot bar. Guess what was just brought out to the hot bar? Signature South Carolina barbecued pork roast. The very food I had PLANNED ON EATING as soon as I arrived prior to my enlightenment. It smelled so good. Yum. Memories of my mom making pork roast for me on my birthday came flooding back. It held a warm and delicious place in my heart. Comfort called my name! OK. Slight modification: I am a vegan that occasionally eats fresh pork roast. That's OK, right? The dilemma of this new vegan that occasionally eats pork roast was that I had filled up my plate already with salad. I quickly solved this vexing issue by pushing some salad aside on my plate and slapping down a piece of pork roast

Chapter 8 – This is the definition of a Turning Point—

in the small void. Normally, I would have bumped my elbow on the salad bar on the way to the hot bar and loaded my entire plate up with pork roast. I put maybe only 10% of the meat on my plate as I would normally eat.

We sat down. Previous meat-eater Bruce would have ravenously tucked into a plate of barbequed animal flesh, but I reminded myself that I WAS a vegan that occasionally ate pork roast, so I ate the BIG salad first. I was scared and anxious, but I sucked down those veggies, and for the first time in my life, I had given my body the primary food it was designed to eat (plants), and it responded as nature designed it to: I was full.

This was a light bulb moment: I quickly mapped out how I would systematically introduce every vegetable imaginable into my diet at every meal. The key to my success in this radical behavioral shift was what I call the "Guilty Pleasure." I realized I could keep the feeling of deprivation at bay while making this transition by simply having a very small portion on my plate of the foods that I loved but now knew were disease-promoting. My good ole comfort friend, Mr. Pork Roast, was there with me the whole time while I learned to eat what I now know is the best diet for human health AND for men dealing with PC. Within a week (I was very determined), that "Guilty Pleasure" of animal flesh simply did not make it to my plate. I was feeling SO MUCH BETTER physically eating this way; the lure of experiencing real health made giving up the foods I had eaten my whole life much easier. And I now know these foods were major contributors to my cancer development.

Summary

1. You have to EAT the food to obtain the health benefits.
2. Deprivation leads to failure. If you need a "guilty pleasure," put a small portion of whatever it is on your plate and eat it last, knowing that this food does not support your health. Drop it off the plate as soon as possible.
3. As your taste buds adapt, you will begin to enjoy this new way of eating. You will start to feel better and let the guilty pleasure fall off your plate.

CHAPTER 9
THE DIAGNOSIS

You hear the word "cancer," and you think it is a death sentence. In fact, the shock is the biggest thing about a diagnosis of cancer.

— Clare Balding

The medical proof of the power of transitioning to eating a Whole-Food, Plant-Based Diet (WFPBD) came only six weeks later with a comprehensive blood panel. In just six weeks of eating primarily fruits, vegetables, grains, nuts, and seeds, I had lost close to 10 pounds, my triglycerides had dropped down to acceptable levels, and my total cholesterol went from 276 to 185. Almost a 100-point drop in six weeks. I proved to myself as my own lab rat that Dr. Campbell was telling the truth. Food is more powerful than drugs in bringing down cholesterol. I was stunned again and very proud as I was also becoming much better at selecting and enjoying healthy food. I made an appointment with my doc, printed the blood panel summary, and marched into his office. "Look," I said, "a 100-point drop in cholesterol just by changing what I eat, and with no drugs." He scanned the report, looked up at me over his reading glasses and said, "Great job, but your PSA is 5.2 which is considered elevated. I want you to see a urologist."

WHAT? I am trying to prove a point here. I don't even know what PSA IS!

"What's PSA?" I ask. And the journey begins……

You probably experienced a very similar situation. The door had just creaked open to a big world of FEAR that I was not familiar with. Suddenly, my data-driven rational mind began to be taken over by an irrational, scattered new emotion: FEAR.

I went into the urologist's office the next day. He does a quick digital rectal exam, and I can see it in his eyes. "We need to do a biopsy. I think you may have a problem."

My wonderful world was beginning to crumble. The biopsy was the next day. FEAR was now top dog in every thought, decision, and lack of decisions that I made. The mistake, which I had no control over, was letting fear rule ALL of my decision making. I simply did not have the tools to battle it.

"This is not going to kill you." I did hear that as Mindy and I sat in the urologist's office that afternoon. Pretty much everything else was a blur of a bad dream.

Here are your options: Do nothing (not recommended by the urologist), radiation (effective, but not a

Chapter 9 – The Diagnosis

guarantee), or robotic surgery to remove the prostate. He, of course, was recommending surgery to "cure" me. My frantic brain quickly latched onto the word "cure," and I made my mind up right then and there that I was going to have surgery. There was simply no way my mind could step back, objectively analyze the situation, and then make a rational, reasoned decision. "I want it out. I want it out RIGHT NOW!" My experience with cancer up to this point was watching my cousin die in her mid-thirties of tongue cancer, followed by Mindy's mom being overtaken by pancreatic cancer at 69. My brain was not in the mood to negotiate, and it said, "Take it out."

In retrospect, I do believe that we would have made the same decision under more rational, mindful circumstances. The initial biopsy results suggested a T2a stage with 11 cores taken, 2 positive, indicative it contained cancer within the prostate's left side. All indications at that time did point to surgery as probably the best (medical) route. But we still made the rookie PC mistake of making a critical, life-changing decision, based on fear, not research. My urologist was an excellent practitioner, experienced with robotic surgery, very smart, and had a great reputation. But he was a urologist, and any urologist is going to lean towards surgery because that's what they know, and at the time, surgery was considered "The Gold Standard" of prostate cancer treatment.

What I SHOULD have done was gone home and begin doing research into treatments, but there was simply no way I could do this. I was completely mentally and emotionally incapacitated. When the doc told me we needed to wait six weeks for my prostate to heal from the biopsy, prior to surgery, I almost exploded. I wanted to be wheeled into the operating room RIGHT NOW. Six weeks??? That was the worst six weeks in my life. I had no tools to deal with what was happening to me. Death by cancer felt much closer than it was.

Mindy's Perspective

Waiting for the results of the biopsy was excruciating. In retrospect, waiting for everything this past nine years has been the hardest part of the journey. As I mentioned earlier, my role is to provide care. To me, that means to FIX. I had lost my mom years before to pancreatic cancer, and I knew all too well what an ugly word cancer was. How could this be happening? The week before we found out about Bruce's cancer, I proclaimed to Bruce that I couldn't think of a more perfect life. And now this. I had no suggestions, and I had no idea of the proper course of action to take. The doctor seemed competent, and he had come with glowing reviews. I didn't think a second opinion was warranted, and I just wanted Bruce to feel content with his

Chapter 9 – The Diagnosis

decision. "Our decision," he kept reminding me. At that point though, I really felt it was his decision as it was his body and his cancer. As you will find out, that way of thinking quickly changed as this cancer that Bruce has is our disease, our journey, and all decisions are made as a team. At the time, however, the gravity of the journey hadn't settled in. How could it? I just thought that the prostate will be removed, and all of this will be behind us. My job is to just keep Bruce preoccupied until it gets sucked out of him with that robot thingy. Little did I know that the journey had just begun.

Non-negotiable: After a diagnosis like this one, never go to a doctor's appointment without a loved one and/or caregiver. Slow down, take your time, find a PC specialist, investigate all of your options with a rational partner/caregiver, and then make your decision. DON'T LET FEAR MAKE DECISIONS FOR YOU! I can't emphasize this enough. You HAVE enough time to sort through this first decision, and it's going to be the most important one you make.

The one coping tool I DID have was alcohol. I was already drinking too much—every night. And now it was the only hammer I had available to knock myself unconscious in the evenings to try to sleep. I was still a new vegan. Great news, Bruce! Gin is VEGAN! No one told me to stop drinking, so I continued to soldier on with the martinis. I was still in the "pre-contemplative stage" of behavioral change as it relates to alcohol. I was now a vegan who was drinking WAY too much and using it as a tool to blunt the pain and fear that comes along with emotional collapse. Not good.

Summary

1. Don't let fear rule your decision making. Take your time and do your research
2. Include the people closest to you in this unventured territory to assist you in mapping your journey forward.
3. Alcohol is not the way to deal with stress and anxiety. Get help if you need it now. Covered in detail later in the book.

CHAPTER 10
SURGERY AND RADIATION—
JANUARY 2012

Be proud of your scars. Those are the badges you've earned from the challenges of life.

— Anonymous

It was a cold and rainy January day in Santa Cruz. Seven hours of robotic surgery later, I woke up in the recovery room in extreme pain. I was given an additional dose of morphine or whatever and wheeled off to my mandatory one-night stay in the hospital. There I was, in my room with Mindy, post-surgery. (I am ashamed of this story, but it's true, and I gotta tell it.) It was around 5:00 p.m. (the time of day is one of the main triggers of bad behaviors that become habits). I am numbed up with opiates, and…. like a Pavlovian dog…. I know it's time for a…. martini. Let's face it; it was a long and stressful day! Let's suspend the fact that I was drugged unconscious for most of it! It was 5 p.m., and I have a martini at 5 p.m. Every day. Period. I called our oldest son, Drew, who was at our house, and asked him to make me a martini and bring it to me in my hospital room (for some crazy reason, there was no open bar inside the hospital, which surprises me because you can sure load up on cancer and heart disease-promoting food inside the very institution that is trying to help mitigate the very same diseases; but that's another whole story).

Anyway, there I am in my bed, sipping a very dry gin martini while I have my post-surgery briefing with my urologist. He dismissed my sipping a martini while still high on morphine and told me the surgery had gone very well. He posited that I was in an elevated pain situation because "I was so skinny, there just wasn't a lot of room to navigate robots and knives in my abdomen.

Three days later, the final pathology report came back: Seminal vesical invasion and a positive margin to boot—80% of the prostate gland contained cancer. The only glimmer of positive news was my Gleason score 7(3+4). Slower growing, I was told. Slower Growing? I'm 53 years old, and cancer has already taken over most of my prostate and was beginning to leave the prostate bed in search of additional homes in my body. I cannot describe the panic and anxiety that enveloped me, but I am sure some of you probably can relate.

The good news was I was up and mobile within two days after surgery, and about three days after that, I was in the water attempting to surf again.

I was determined to get back into surf shape as quickly as possible. I work out every day and surf whenever I can. Exercise and physical activity have always come easy for me because I love the feeling of physical exertion. It's essential to stay as active as possible post diagnosis and post treatment. It's easy for me, but I know how difficult it can be to begin an exercise regime in your 50s, 60s, and 70s if you haven't made a habit of it. It's not as difficult as you might think. It's honestly as easy as stepping out your front door and walking around the neighborhood at a comfortable brisk pace EVERY DAY for at least 20 minutes. I could write an entire book on the benefits of exercise for cancer patients. In summary, the entire global cancer medical treatment community is in agreement: Exercise is a critical component for cancer therapy and recovery. According to Harvard Health Publishing, The Clinical Oncology Society of Australia (COSA) became the first national cancer center to issue formal guidelines that recommend exercise as a part of ALL cancer treatments. You don't need a gym membership or fancy equipment. Get up, put on some comfy shoes, and walk briskly around the block. If you feel OK, do it again! If you're winded, try jogging a few steps and increase as you adapt. It's really that simple.[1]

I was pretty much back physically from the surgery within a few weeks, but just two months later, my post-surgery PSA was 0.03 ng/ml. NOT undetectable as it should be after surgery. Grrrr. That spring, just four months post-surgery, my urologist referred me to a local radiation oncologist. He explained to us that the plan was to proceed with daily salvage external beam radiation therapy (EBRT) to my prostate bed to "clean up what was left of the cancer." Here again, FEAR was my primary decision-maker. I didn't do any research or talk to anyone else. We agreed and began EBRT radiation therapy to my prostate bed every day during the work week for six weeks. Now, at this point, you need to realize that I had made nutritional research my full-time job, and I began the eCornell (Cornell University's online education platform) Plant-Based Certification Course created by Dr. Campbell himself. I was quickly becoming very knowledgeable about evidence-based nutritional science. I had already radically changed my eating behavior and was a true plant-based eater at this point. And dare I say an "emerging" enthusiast on evidenced-based nutrition.

Radiation

About one-and-a-half weeks into my adjuvant prostate bed EBRT in the early summer of 2012, I was in the waiting room with probably 13 people, most of whom were women with headscarves on probably because of the combo radiation and chemo treatment they were receiving. One of the nurses, who was extremely obese, like most doctors' office employees I have met, comes into the waiting room with a giant tray full of... DONUTS. Are you kidding me? Donuts served in a radiation waiting room full of people just like me who ended up in here BECAUSE of lifelong poor diets? I just couldn't believe it. I mentioned this to my new radiation oncologist who, again, just like every doctor I had met with or spoken to regarding my cancer up to this point, had little understanding of the overwhelming scientific evidence of the relationship of fatty, fried, empty-calorie foods, and the development of cancer. Just like all the other doctors I had encountered so far in my PC journey, this radiation oncologist dismissed the incident, letting me know that his patients needed a little treat due to their unfortunate situation. Ugg again. That's all I can say.

Anyway, I endured the six-week protocol without complications or side-effects. And again, after completion of this treatment, my PSA went.... UP. From 0.04 to 0.05. The radiation oncologist explained the radiation PSA "bump" theory to me, but it was of little solace, as over the next few months, my PSA continued its upward trend. I was feeling beat down again and beginning to lose hope.

Summary

1. Make a commitment to stay on a healthy eating and movement routine.
2. Learn everything you can about PC and what all the numbers mean; don't hide from it!
3. Educate yourself on what you can do to mitigate the side effects of treatment.

CHAPTER 11
MY FIRST BREAKDOWN IN NYC 2013

Crying is how your heart speaks when your lips can't explain the pain you feel.

— Anonymous

The ECA (East Coast Alliance for Aerobic & Fitness Professionals, in New York State) holds a convention at the Marriott Marquis (https://www.marriott.com/hotels/travel/sfodt-san-francisco-marriott-marquis/) in Times Square every year. This year, Mindy and I have a booth to sell products, and we are also featured speakers. I was now on the lecture circuit at these conferences, and I loved it. Nutrition found me and pulled me in. It was the best thing that ever happened to me, other than marrying my wife and having three awesome kids. But here I was, at the Marriott, trying to focus on my presentations, make money at the booth, and grapple with the fact that my PSA was on the rise again. I was still drinking way too much. (When lecturing, I always told my audience that alcohol was plant-based.) The combination of rising PSA, business pressures, constant plane travel, and FEAR of the unknown pushed me into a realm that I had never known before—emotional breakdown.

I was alone in our hotel room (Mindy was teaching an evening class), and my fear took over. I just could not see a way out of my horrible dilemma. I took a long shower, and ended up curled up naked like a baby, crying uncontrollably on the floor. This is what Mindy got to see and experience when she walked into our room. I honestly thought I was completely losing it mentally. It was an ugly, cathartic experience. This was letting go emotionally and completely for the first time in my life. The scene was made worse by the fact that I HATED (and still do) what I was putting my family through and Mindy in particular. I honestly thought it might be best if I removed myself and my misery from my family. Just move somewhere where they would not have to suffer my deep pain. I cried myself to sleep like a child.

I woke up the next day, and I felt, well, better! A lifelong weight felt as if it had been lifted from me—emotional suppression. Get rid of it. It will kill you in the long run!

My advice to you: Have a breakdown and let yourself cry like a baby. You will be a better person for it. This has been an unexpected gift of cancer for me. Years of controlling and suppressing emotions is a really bad idea. Cancer or not, learn, hell, LET yourself be emotional. Doing this has completely changed my life and how I view it. Too many of us men have grown up figuring out (no one ever taught us how; it's just implied)

Chapter 11 – My First Breakdown in NYC 2013

that society expects us to maintain a neutral, detached, emotional state regardless of the situation. That's just how it was, and still is, and it is complete bullshit. My life, even with cancer, has become SO MUCH more fulfilling and meaningful since I learned to let go emotionally with the people I care about most. It's beyond better. I would go so far as to say that living an emotionally walled-off life like I had my entire life up to this point is simply WRONG.

Now there is a fine line between becoming emotionally available and feeling sorry for yourself. I went through the "poor me" stage after diagnosis. It probably lasted up until my first emotional breakdown. I don't know how to avoid the "poor me" stage, and maybe you can't, but get through it as fast as possible. Getting from "poor me" to "I am taking charge of my health and my life and to hell with anything or anyone who stands in my way" should happen as quickly as possible. Don't wallow longer than needed in the "poor me" stage. It was at this point in my journey that I accepted that my lifestyle and eating habits were strongly correlated with my cancer development and progression. And in addition, I KNEW, from all my research, that I may not be able to control my outcome, but I certainly DO have tremendous power to influence it through mindfulness, meditation, letting go, and DIET!

I was in the "poor me" stage way too long. Bone up, cry like a baby, and then BE A MAN! But be a man with emotion.

With my PSA rising, my urologist now recommended I make an appointment with a leading PC research scientist at UCSF. Here we go again. It's the spring of 2013, and my PSA is now 1.20, and another doctor enters my world. With impressive credentials, he was presently recruiting patients for a clinical trial of a new derivative hormone therapy treatment. From the first meeting, my impression was that this doctor and his team were more concerned with having me participate in his clinical trial than he was interested in my personal situation. I asked him if he was aware of Dr. Dean Ornish's randomized controlled trials at UCSF using a vegan diet to slow the growth of early-stage prostate cancer. Nope. Any nutritional recommendations? Nope. He mentioned that he had "heard" pomegranate juice might be beneficial. That's it. I then asked him if he had any recommendations for calming the anxiety and stress that I was experiencing on a daily basis. YES! Here is a prescription for Xanax. Did I mention I have an addictive personality? I started taking it, and it did help lower my stress, and I thought I might be stabilizing emotionally. But according to Mindy, the drug rendered me a little... numb emotionally. I used it for about two months straight and then ditched it in favor of.... cannabis. More on this later.

Summary

1. Come to terms with your situation emotionally.

Chapter 11 – My First Breakdown in NYC 2013

2. Allow yourself to collapse and cry.
3. The lowest lows can give way to the highest highs if you open up emotionally with the ones you love the most.

CHAPTER 12
MORE DOCS AND THE BEACH HOUSE – SPRING OF 2013

Time waits for no one.

— Folklore

Mindy and I love to ride bikes. We also love to go to open houses as we consider ourselves good interior designers. We lived in the foothills of Santa Cruz a few miles from the ocean, and we always talked about buying a "cottage" on the beach when we retired, but I never seriously thought it was a possibility because a house on the beach in this part of California was always way out of reach financially for us, or so I thought. Nothing like the realization that life is VERY short to make bold moves.

We were riding our bikes on West Cliff Drive—a stunningly beautiful oceanfront path that meanders by several of my favorite surf spots, including Steamer Lane in Santa Cruz. Every time I went surfing, which was most days in the fall and winter, I would have to put all of my surf gear in my car and drive 15 minutes down to the beach. Not a terrible trek by any means, but living at the beach would be better! Anyway, we are cruising on our bikes, and Mindy stops in front of an open house sign and said we should go check it out. I just wanted to go on a bike ride and check the surf. I knew there was no way we could afford ANY house that close to the beach. I put up a mild protest, but Mindy persisted, so I turned around, and we headed to the open house.

When we rode up, we could tell the place was in complete shambles and had not been occupied for at least a few years. There was a guy sleeping in a lawn chair in front of the house. He was the next-door neighbor and was standing in for the realtor who was supposed to be holding the open house. You could tell right away that he didn't expect us to be interested. But he was charming and funny. We went in. What a disaster. Old and mold and more old and mold. What I did notice immediately was that there was a nice peek of the ocean out of each of the downstairs windows. But still a hot mess of a house. We almost turned around to leave when Mindy saw narrow stairs and up we went.

As soon as I reached the top of the stairs, a stunning view of the Santa Cruz Boardwalk, the 100-year-old Santa Cruz wharf, and pretty much the entire Monterey Bay revealed itself through giant windows. The whole top floor was nothing but windows and views of whales and surfers and dolphins and surf and pretty much everything I loved about the ocean. The upstairs itself was a WRECK as well. The neighbor said that hundreds of people had paraded through the house, but none could even begin to grasp how to remodel. We saw the potential immediately and made an offer that night. We closed, moved in, and began a massive remodeling project that turned that old beater into a stunning modern home with spectacular views. I love that house. WE love that house.

Mindy's Perspective

The best thing you both can do for the two of you is to love where you live and live where you love. As Bruce mentioned, it had always been our dream to live at the beach. But "someday, maybe" always got in the way. Everything up until recently was status quo, so better stay put. Well, Bruce's cancer wasn't staying put, so neither would we. I knew that if I got Bruce to the beach, his whole world would change. He could see the ocean every day. He could walk just around the corner to his favorite surf spot. And all of that would be an upside, net positive toward health. Also, it gave Bruce much to focus on besides cancer and nutrition research. Diving too often into the weeds of research can be debilitating to say the least, and I was grateful for this distraction. Our remodel was massive and all-consuming. Just what Bruce needed. And after it was done, we had our dream house in our dream location. That "someday, maybe" had become reality.

Summary

1. Identify what your ideal life looks like and what really brings you happiness.

2. Do whatever it takes to turn your dreams into reality.
3. You may never see your dreams come true if you don't act now.

CHAPTER 13
ALTERNATIVE TREATMENTS

The greatest medicine of all is to teach people how not to use it.

— Hippocrates

In late 2013, I was on a mission to investigate every alternative PC treatment available. First up: Budwig Diet. The Budwig dietary intervention for PC is as follows: No clinical research or data that I was able to locate. I didn't care. It was easy to try and quite delicious. Basically, you mix flax oil with cottage cheese and eat it. This was a big departure from the strict vegan diet I was following, but what the hell. I did the Budwig diet for about a month, but it had no impact on my rising PSA. Budwig, done. I suppose you could give it a try, but I would recommend a pass. Why load up on liquid processed plant fat and cow's milk? Both are implicated in chronic disease and PC specifically.

I then found the Rick Simpson website. I was a regular user of cannabis throughout college and a few years after that, but I gave it up in my late 20s. And what did I do when I gave up cannabis? I started drinking more! As

I mentioned earlier, drinking was encouraged in my career position; it was socially acceptable, and I loved it. I am sure it was also feeding my cancer's growth along with a meat-centered, fatty, processed food diet. At this point, medical cannabis was legal in California (thank you, California!). The Simpson site had great testimonials about both Rick Simpson and others curing themselves of advanced PC by simply orally consuming 60 grams of THC (tetrahydrocannabinol) heavy cannabis oil in 90 days. 60 grams in 90 days? WHAT? That's a tall order, but I was going to give it a go.

I got my medical cannabis card and drove to the only dispensary that sold the Rick Simpson Oil (RSO) product in San Jose. I bought 60 grams of the oil and drove home. I had not used any cannabis for at least 20 years. Per the instructions, I started out ingesting orally, a small rice-size dot of the oil. No problem, I thought. I know my weed. Uh, no, I didn't. Two hours later, I was SLAMMED STONED. I was completely toasted. The next day, I told Mindy that I did not think I could go through with the entire protocol because it would render me stupid and catatonic for three months, and I had a business to run and work to do. What I DID notice was that I actually felt great the next day. No headache, no hangover, and actually a lot of energy. Mr. Simpson assured me on his website that I would quickly build up a tolerance to the THC, so I decided to proceed. I doubled the dosage the next day, and the next. Each successive day, even with the increased dosage, I was adapting. I

Chapter 13 – Alternative Treatments

could function for most of the day at work. I'd take the dosage in the early afternoon, and then, well, I wasn't much good to anybody a few hours later, but I actually was feeling pretty damn good. The major change to my behavior during that experience was that I fell asleep at around eight or nine o'clock and slept for at least nine to ten hours. For the first time since my diagnosis, I was sleeping comfortably and thoroughly through the night without waking up with anxiety and fear. And I felt great the next day. I completed this crazy, scientifically undocumented protocol in less than 80 days. I was a star student! Did it change my PSA velocity or trajectory? No. But it did allow me, for the first time since this whole PC journey, to sleep without interruption. Although I gave up on the Rick Simpson treatment to "cure" me, I did not stop using cannabis.

Mindy's Perspective

Living with cancer is tough stuff, and as caregivers, we have no idea what our loved one is emotionally dealing with on a minute-by-minute basis. Bruce used alcohol, and later, an anti-depressant drug to help with his anxiety. Both had side-effects that were ugly. Cannabis offered Bruce, for the first time since being diagnosed, a restful night's sleep with no hangover the next day. Don't let outdated judgement cloud what cannabis can do to help mitigate the side effects of a cancer diagnosis.

Summary

1. Don't let social stigma or outdated laws or beliefs stand in the way of exploring alternative treatment—especially for stress and anxiety reduction.
2. If you do choose to try alternative treatments like cannabis, make sure to share all information with your caregiver and your doctor/oncologist so that they can best help you.
3. Cannabis has been a powerful tool for me personally.

CHAPTER 14
THE BOOK, *FEAR: ESSENTIAL WISDOM FOR GETTING THROUGH THE STORM,* AND THE BEGINNING OF MY MEDITATION PRACTICE

The only way to ease our fear and be truly happy is to acknowledge our fear and look deeply at its source. Instead of trying to escape from our fear, we can invite it up to our awareness and look at it clearly and deeply.

— Thich Nhat Hanh

Christmas 2013 was not pleasant. It seems like every Christmas since being diagnosed, I end up getting blood work done and getting the results when my whole family is together for special occasions and holidays. Wham. Another rise in PSA, my predictable fuming frustration and anger, my family consoling me (this has to be getting old for them), and then within 24 to 48 hours, acceptance, and planning next steps with resolve. This is such a repeating pattern that I knew I had to have some help dealing with it emotionally. How can this go on for the rest of my life? Every month another blood test with usually lousy results. Sometimes it almost feels like I am watching a big countdown clock to my death. Everyone has this clock, but those of us dealing with long term PC have a Big Ben in their head with a flashing neon Las Vegas sign: Your cancer is growing, and you are getting closer to the end. Buy a beach house!

Anyway, my oldest son's girlfriend at the time bought me a book (thank you, Ellie!) as a gift and left it for me on the coffee table. I was in my room in a "poor me" state of mind and feeling sorry for myself after receiving my last blood test. The book was entitled *FEAR: Essential Wisdom for Getting Through the Storm* by Thich Nhat Hanh. The title of THIS book should be: *Fear and How to Manage It.* I was in a raw state and read the entire book. Buy the book!! Thich Nhat Hanh has taught me many things, but the most important is that everyone suffers, and the best way to relieve suffering is to acknowledge it and help others who are suffering. He elegantly explains that none of us can hide from our suffering, and when trying to through media, consumption, consumerism, drugs, or materialistic means, it only makes the situation worse. The key is in HOW we deal with our suffering.

This was when I began my meditation practice that has now become an integral part of my life and my cancer therapy. Thich Nhat Hanh showed me, through meditation, how to bring the suffering into my mind on

PURPOSE and let my mind dwell on it and then LET IT GO. The power of meditation is real, and it has become my go-to power tool in helping me deal with anxiety and FEAR. What's the downside of giving it a try? None. How much does it cost? It's FREE.

For that matter, everything that I have implemented in my life (low-fat, whole food, plant-based diet/ meditation/exercise) is in this book, and it is FREE with no negative side effects. What's the downside of giving meditation a try? NONE. Upside? Enlightenment, reduction of anxiety and fear, a sense of overall well-being, and feeling happier. Science supports these upsides as well.

In 2017, the American Society of Clinical Oncology (ASCO) published a small pilot study from Northwestern University where men on active surveillance were randomized to either mindfulness (n = 24) or an attention control arm (n = 19) and completed self-reported measures of prostate cancer anxiety, uncertainty intolerance, global quality of life, mindfulness, and posttraumatic growth at baseline, eight weeks, six months, and twelve months. The participants in the mindfulness arm demonstrated significant decreases in prostate cancer anxiety and uncertainty intolerance, and significant increases in mindfulness, global mental health, and posttraumatic growth. Posttraumatic growth was shown to significantly increase over time for men in the treatment group. Mindfulness training has the potential to help men cope more effectively with some of the stressors and uncertainties associated with active surveillance and just dealing with it in general.[1]

Mindy's Perspective

Bruce and I started our meditation journey with the 21-day challenge with Deepak Chopra. Meditation is an interesting activity because when you first start, you don't know what you are doing, and for some reason, every skin surface starts to itch, and any thought that you had ever thought in your life comes popping into your brain for no good reason at all. The 21-day meditation challenge focused on guided meditation—a practitioner leads you down a thoughtful path and then leaves you with your own thoughts and then guides you back.

All I can say is "wow." I don't know when I have ever cried so much or seen Bruce cry so much. These mindful nudges in the guided meditations opened doors for us that we didn't even know were within us, let alone were closed tight prior to meditation. Mindful meditation has been a saving grace for both of us. We each have our own favorite way to practice—Bruce now uses a head sling and lies on the floor. That way doesn't work for me because I would immediately fall asleep. I usually sit or run. Sometimes the meditation lasts for two minutes or twenty. No right or wrong way. The beauty of meditation is that it is always available and always free. And did I mention, "Meditation is a WOW."

Summary

1. FEAR sucks. You must develop a strategy for dealing with constant low-level fear and anxiety—it is not going to go away, so learn how to manage it, not run from it. For most men with recurrent PC, it is all about the blood test.
2. Meditation is my powerful tool for managing my FEAR and anxiety.
3. Download one of the free apps (https://thejoywithin.org/authors/deepak-chopra/abundance-meditation-challenge) on the internet (like this one from Deepak Chopra).

CHAPTER 15
I LOVE MARTINIS!

Reality is an illusion that occurs because of a lack of alcohol.

— W. C. Fields

At this point, for the next several months, we watched my PSA continue to rise, reaching 1.40 in the summer of 2015. In addition to being scared, frustrated, and angry, I made the decision that I was not going to work with a medical practice or doctors that at least did not acknowledge or understand the importance of evidence-based nutrition in the development and treatment of the most common cancers in our country. In early 2015, I contacted Dr. Mark Renneker, a board certified family physician who is now a medical advocate for people with cancer and other serious medical conditions. I wish I had done this right after finding out I had PC, but no dwelling on the past. Move forward. Keep moving. I sent Dr. R all of my records and family history that he had requested and scheduled a phone consultation.

Mindy and I were at our new kitchen counter at our newly remodeled house on the beach (it's awesome) waiting for our five p.m. phone consultation with one of the most well-respected oncologists I could find. Turns out, he is also a legendary big-wave surfer from San Francisco, which just added to his stature as far as I was concerned. The first 20 minutes of the phone consult was a recap of my family history, tumor biopsy, and current health. I got an A+ for my diet, and I was thrilled about the fact that I had finally found a doctor who understood the importance of plant-based eating for cancer recovery. Then it came. It went something like this:

Dr. R: "I noticed on the questionnaire you filled out for me that you drink alcohol. Can you tell me about that?"

Me thinking: *Why in the hell is this guy asking me about my alcohol consumption? I knew I was drinking too much but was still able to convince myself that this was not an issue!*

Me saying: "Uh, well, yeah. Of course, I have a drink in the evening to unwind. It's stressful running your burgeoning new business AND dealing with PC. No big deal."

Dr. R: "No big deal? What time of day do you drink?"

Me: "Evenings mostly. Occasional beer at lunch or during the day on the weekends."

Dr. R: "What do you drink?"

Chapter 15 – I Love Martinis!

Me: "Vodka martinis." (I had convinced myself that vodka has some magical property that made it a better choice than other hard alcohol.)

Dr. R: "Does Mindy drink?"

Me: "Yes, wine in the evening."

Dr. R: "Do you drink wine as well as martini's?"

Me: "Well, uh, yeah, sometimes" (thinking: Please let's move on to another subject).

Dr. R: "How many glasses of wine? How many martini's?"

And on and on, drilling down to where I did NOT want to be drilled. I was feeling pinned to the wall by my newfound consultant, and he was not going to let this go. After about 10 miserable and very expensive minutes discussing my alcohol use (read abuse), I could see the writing on the wall, and I knew what was coming. I wanted to run away, but I couldn't. And to top it off, this was all happening at 5:30 p.m., when the Pavlovian martini bell was beginning to chime loudly in my head. It was time to start drinking!

At the end of this telephone inquisition, and after what seemed like an eternal pause of silence (probably less than 10 seconds), Dr. R said, and I'll never forget, "Bruce, you are a fucking idiot! Quit drinking. NOW." No mincing of words here. Nothing like candid observation and advice from someone you paid a lot of money to and have tremendous respect for. The rest of the consultation was also very important and life-changing (more below), but I don't think anything else was really registering for me. I hung up the phone, and Mindy and I stared at each other. I did not realize it at the time, but I had just moved from the "pre-contemplation" stage of behavioral change to the "take action" state of behavioral change with alcohol. No other doctor had asked me about my drinking habits up until this point.

I grabbed the 1.5 liters of Costco Stolichnaya vodka from the freezer. I made a very LARGE martini, drank it, then I poured the rest of the bottle down the drain of my kitchen sink. After 20 some odd years of a nightly highball, or two, or three, that consultation with Dr. R was the trigger that pulled me out of alcohol abuse denial. Better late than never! I quit. Cold turkey. We all have certain triggers that will finally unlock the chains of addiction and bad habits, and this was mine. I would highly recommend doing some soul searching to figure out what your triggers are if you are trying to improve your health and save yourself from cancer.

Since giving up the hard stuff, I sleep better, and I wake up feeling energized and ready for the day. Dr. R was right. I WAS a fucking idiot! I am so glad he called me on it, and I finally admitted it to myself.

Honestly, almost all books on nutrition have a chapter on alcohol. I know, because I have read most of them! But in my 52 years of lounging in the pre-contemplation stage of behavioral change as it relates to alcohol, I would always flip by the pages describing the detriments of drinking to get to the next section. I knew it

Chapter 15 – I Love Martinis!

was a problem for me deep in my brain somewhere; I just did not want to confront it. If you drink and have PC, confront it. We all love good news about our bad habits, but a recent meta-analysis from the University of Washington School of Medicine sealed the deal for me. The research summary, which was a part of the "Global Burden of Disease Study" (GBD) and published in *The Lancet,* looked at levels of alcohol use and its health effects in 195 countries, including the UK, between 1990 and 2016. Analyzing data from 15 to 95-year-olds, the researchers compared people who did not drink at all with those who had one alcoholic drink a day. They found that out of 100,000 non-drinkers, less than one percent would develop an alcohol-related health problem such as cancer or suffer an injury. The researchers summarize, "There is no safe level of drinking alcohol." It shows that in 2016, nearly three million deaths globally were attributed to alcohol use.[1]

The optimum amount of alcohol for humans: ZERO. The Optimum alcohol consumption for cancer care: ZERO. I get it if you like to drink. I LOVE alcohol. I still have a glass of wine with dinner occasionally when I know it's probably better to pass. But something motivates me even more: I love being alive and thriving. Don't convince yourself you are doing something healthy by drinking wine or any other alcoholic beverage. If you are battling cancer, you are better off without it. Period.

~ ~ ~

Expert Analysis—Dr. Michael Klaper

> Alcohol is Evil, with a capital "E." It knocks down your immune cells' ability to eat up cancer germs and cancer cells. The more you drink, the higher the cancer risk, and that's the last thing you need right now. You want your immune system as sober as possible.

Every day at 5:30 p.m., the martini bell still rings in my head, but I have learned to REPLACE my bad habit with a good one. I love cooking, and I could easily live the rest of my life in my kitchen. Part of my dinner prep ritual, like many, was to pour myself a hefty drink and get started. I do the same thing now, but instead of pouring myself a martini, I make myself a cup of hibiscus tea with a slice of dried ginger and ginseng, with a slice of lemon. It's a time-consuming goofy ritual, JUST LIKE MAKING A BEAUTIFUL MARTINI. I still have a ritual, but now it's a healthy one. The urge to imbibe is still there, but once I have finished dinner, the desire, the NEED for alcohol, is gone.

But not to minimize or downplay the rest of the discussion with Dr. R. For the first time, I really felt like I was taking control of my health and my PC treatment strategy. I was beginning to take charge, and I would make my own decisions about how to proceed. The best advice Dr. R gave me other than to stop poisoning myself with alcohol was to reach out to other medical specialists in

Chapter 15 – I Love Martinis!

the field and get a second and third opinion. He pointed us in the direction of Dr. Mark Scholz and his team of oncologists at Prostate Oncology Specialists (PROS) in Marina Del Rey as they were on the leading edge of prostate cancer treatment. He also said I could benefit from a full day personal consultation at the Block Medical Center in Chicago, headed up by Dr. Keith Block.

We contacted PROS and the Block Center for Integrative Oncology and made an appointment with both. I was determined to be patient and review all of my options rationally this time.

Mindy's Perspective

Under extreme stress, Bruce cannot cope well with logistics, navigating the details. This is where I step in. I make the appointments; I talk to the nurses; I order the lab tests and request the medications. Bruce handles a lot, but when I can take over and wade through some of the details that make Bruce go a little crazy, it is the least I can do. Do not fault the patient for not being able to handle the minor details. They have a lot going on inside that we can't even comprehend. The job of cancer maintenance takes its toll, and in our case, as caregivers, it is important for the caregiver to be the logistics master.

This topic also brings me to another very important subject. Knowledge is empowering and shows others you are able to sit at the same table. Early on in the game, I didn't want to know the details of Bruce's stage of cancer as I was afraid of what that might entail. I didn't want to address the severity of the stats. I always knew when Bruce was doing research, as his mood became dark, and there was nothing I could do. He would shake his head and say, "Min, it isn't good. My chances aren't good for my stage of cancer. The stats aren't in my favor." I would remind him that he wasn't a stat. Manage your health and not your numbers. But again, these are but words.

I bought myself a necklace that has the word HOPE engraved in it, and I wear it every day. This is what we all have—HOPE. And I do believe that those who are hopeful have better outcomes than those who are not hopeful. However, I have to come to the realization that hope doesn't manage the day-to-day operations. I had to know the details and become an expert myself on Bruce's cancer if I was to help him in every way possible. I had to know the PSA numbers and what they mean, remember the dates of procedures and past and current meds, make friends with the staff at the doctors' offices—and be MOMMA BEAR (or Daddy Bear if that pertains to you). Stand up for what you and your loved one needs. No one is in charge of your health but you. This amazing man needs me now more than ever to take the lead.

Summary

1. Seeking out expert opinion is crucial to your decision making. Take your time to find the right team.

Chapter 15 – I Love Martinis!

2. Have an honest personal habit assessment meeting with yourself. Are your life-long habits helping or harming your health? Face your addictions if you have them.
3. Now is the time to surround yourself with friends and not accomplices. Friends want you to be healthy. Accomplices want a friend to party with.

CHAPTER 16
SEARCHING FOR THE RIGHT TEAM

Eighty percent of all choices are based on fear. Most people don't choose what they want; they choose what they think is safe.

— Phil McGraw

Mindy and I flew to Chicago and had the full day intake on a freezing Chicago wintery day in February 2015 at the Block Medical Center of Integrative Oncology. The first session was with a NUTRITIONIST! Oh, food is very important to this team. Every patient that walks into the door at the BMC will be counseled to adopt a whole-food, plant-based diet, while eliminating ALL animal products, including fish, dairy, and eggs. Fortunately, I was already there! Based on my current stats, Dr. Block told us that he believed that my cancer was still at the "curable" stage and suggested I contact a PC medical specialty practice in Florida as they were having great success treating failed RP's (radical prostatectomies) with targeted radiation.

We then flew directly from the Block Center in Chicago to LA, and I had my first intake discussion with Dr. Scholz at PRCO (Prostate Oncology Specialists). I liked the guy from the get-go. He and his team were obviously on top of the latest research on every imaginable PC treatment. THERE WERE FLYERS AT THE RECEPTION DESK ON THE IMPORTANCE OF HEALTHY EATING FOR PROSTATE CANCER! WHAT? Nutrition?

After our initial consultation, Dr. Scholz suggested my first step was to get a prostate-specific membrane antigen (PSMA) gallium positron PET scan, but the only machine currently available at the time was in Europe, and it was not covered by my insurance. What a nightmare insurance is. I touch on this later, but I don't think I need to tell you how scary it is to navigate insurance when dealing with PC. And I did not have company insurance because we were self-employed, which meant that we paid out of pocket around $2000 a month for catastrophic insurance. Anyway, I had a sense of a good fit with POC and Dr. Scholz.

Although I felt I was getting a handle on taking control of my situation, fear was still an overwhelming factor in my decision making. I had a phone consult with this other new doc in Florida while at a hotel in Philadelphia (another fitness conference) the following week. I remember the discussion well because I was sitting next to an elevator shaft at the hotel conference room and was straining to hear every word. I have respect for this doctor, but

Chapter 16 – Searching for the Right Team

looking back, a red flag went up during this phone talk. He could not stop telling me how great his research was, and he was the ONLY ONE PERFORMING THIS TYPE OF RADIATION that he personally had developed WITH GREAT SUCCESS. And yes, he thought he could cure my cancer.

Ah, he said the "CURE" word I wanted to hear SO BADLY. So badly, I made up my mind I was going to proceed. (This was definitely NOT what Dr. Scholz was recommending, and if I could go back, I would have pushed fear out of the way and probably made a different decision). Prior to this treatment, I had an MRI and CAT scan. Both came back negative. No evidence of lymph node or bone involvement. When I spoke with the doc in Florida, he explained to me that my situation was "not unusual" and he was convinced that the PC was in my lymph nodes (even though CAT and MRI indicated otherwise) and that he wanted to go ahead with the eight weeks of radiation to my abdominal lymph nodes coupled with one year of hormone therapy with Lupron and Casodex. Here again, I believe FEAR was my primary tool for decision making. My mind could only hear the word "cure," and it refused to process the red flags.

Mindy and I checked our calendar and booked our summer radiation holiday of 2015 in Florida. How exciting! We were committed. We explained to our office manager that we were going to be in Florida for three months and asked her to do her best to run our business while we were gone, and Mindy would run her end remotely. At this point, I just let go of worrying about what was going to happen with our little company. I simply could not focus on my treatment and our business. This "letting go" was definitely a positive and learning turning point in my journey. Up to this point, I was managing all the financials, marketing, and sales of our little production company. Business was always on my mind. But I was simply unable to continue on like this. I JUST LET IT GO AND ASKED FOR HELP FROM MY BUSINESS TEAM (read: Mindy picked up the slack). What a wonderful relief.

We left our home, office, office manager, and business and headed to Florida for three months in the summer of 2015. To summarize, I should have been much more sensitive to the red flags I was getting, but the combination of FEAR coupled with the possibility of a cure overrode my gut instincts. I now believe that going forward with this procedure without having true identifiable targets (cancer) was a mistake. (I am sure Dr. Scholz would agree.) If I could go back in time, I would have committed to Dr. Scholz and his team and his recommendations, but I didn't.

This bears repeating: DON'T LET FEAR RULE YOUR DECISION MAKING.

Hormone Treatment - Round 1

We showed up in Florida in early May of 2015. I was SCARED of hormone therapy and had been able to avoid it up to this point. I had heard:

Chapter 16 – Searching for the Right Team

- You will lose all interest in sex. WHAT? Sex was one of my core capabilities and a very integral part of my shared life with my very HOT athletic wife. Will she leave me?
- You will lose all of your energy and be tired all the time. That sounds horrible to an athlete, and I live an energetic life.
- You will gain weight and lose muscle mass. Again, a scary thing to hear if you are an active person like me. Not good.

I got my first Lupron shot in that office in Florida in the early summer of 2015. We quickly went back to our rental on the beach and HAD SEX. It all worked, but it was the first day!

I was determined to maintain my physical activities, including sex, and working out for the duration of this radiation treatment in Florida. I weighed myself prior to starting hormone therapy and monitored my weight for the duration of our stay in Florida. I stayed hyper-focused on a low-fat plant-based diet. We rode bikes every day, and I paddled at least a mile on a Costco soft-top surfboard which I bought. Paddle in the morning. Go to radiation. Run or ride bikes in the evening. Every single day. Guess what? The whole process was a breeze with the exception of low-level nausea that was caused by prescription drugs that were part of the protocol. The panic and fear I had nurtured up until that first Lupron shot were completely unfounded. We actually turned it into a two-month vacation that was very pleasant. At the end of the eight weeks, my PSA was undetectable, I had maintained my weight, and my attitude was great, but my interest in sex was zero. More on that to come.

Mindy's Perspective

What Bruce fails to mention is that during these eight weeks, I had us booked at conferences or trainings every weekend. Friday a.m.'s radiation treatments would be followed by a trip to the airport to fly somewhere in the county to one of our speaking commitments. Bruce and I book our schedule at least one year in advance, and when we decided on this treatment option, I had already lined us up for five out of the eight weekends on the road lecturing.

Why didn't I cancel everything and just focus on radiation, laying low, and doing nothing? Two very clear reasons.

First off, the bills don't stop flowing in just because you or your loved one has cancer. Actually, the opposite is true if you are self-employed and much of what you do is "out-of-pocket." With me now handling the finances, I knew that we had to keep working. But the bigger and second reason for pushing through every weekend was that Bruce needed purpose. Bruce is fueled by sharing his passion and his knowledge. He is energized knowing that he has made a difference in someone else's life. Just hunkering down in Florida for eight weeks would have been easy, but it would have in no way been fulfilling for Bruce. It also took his mind off his current situation at least for a little while.

Summary

1. Don't let fear rule your decision making.
2. You have more control of the side effects of cancer treatment than you think. You are not a statistic.
3. Find your purpose. Don't let cancer define who you are.

CHAPTER 17
THERAPY—CANNABIS

Herb is the healing of a nation. Alcohol is the destruction.

— Bob Marley

Cannabis saved my ass during this treatment. As I mentioned, I was taking several prescription drugs in addition to the Casodex and Lupron, and they were giving me a low level of nausea that really sucked my energy. I had brought (smuggled from California) enough of the cannabis oil to last me the duration of the treatment, and I took a little orally at about 4:00 p.m. every day. Nausea—gone. Sleep—easy and eight to nine hours a night. I am not suggesting cannabis for everyone who has prostate cancer because I don't think it's for everybody. What I can tell you is that it has been a lifesaver for me. It was a powerful tool for me dealing with the nausea. It calmed me. It made me hungry, so I would eat, and I was sleeping through the night for the first time since being diagnosed almost three years earlier.

I still swallow (I don't smoke or vape ANYTHING) a small combo of CBD/THC as recommended. Unfortunately, because cannabis is still classified as a

Schedule 1 narcotic by our federal government, professional researchers have historically steered clear of studying the drug. However, there is some very compelling preliminary research demonstrating cannabis's ability to slow the growth of PC. Most importantly though, it allowed me to quit drinking. Did I just swap one addiction for another? Maybe, but I can easily go days without using cannabis (like during fasting) without any withdrawal symptoms.

Dr. Renneker was not opposed to me using cannabis as part of my treatment protocol and commented that it was also my "methadone" for dropping alcohol, and he is absolutely right. I would not dismiss the potential use of this drug as a far better anxiety suppressant than Xanax and certainly alcohol. Don't let social stigma or shame stop you from experimenting with cannabis, especially if you are currently using alcohol or prescription drugs to numb or manage pain, depression, and/or anxiety. There is a very good reason that most states in the US have legalized medical cannabis: Because it helps people.

Bottom line: I use it orally only in a very specific dose and formula (Details in the "What I Do" section). I sleep SO MUCH BETTER with cannabis. I wake up feeling energized, calm, and happy. I'd be delighted to talk with you about my experience. Did it cure my cancer? Nope. Is it slowing down tumor growth? Maybe. Do I ever wake up with a headache and feel like shit? You mean like every morning for 30+ years when

Chapter 17 – Therapy—Cannabis

drinking martinis every night? NO. NEVER. Does it augment my journey to not let fear and anxiety rule my mind? 100%. Finally, let me ask you this: Do you know anyone who has overdosed on cannabis? How many cannabis overdoses have been recorded in the US? None. Ever. It does not happen.

Now let me ask you this: Do you know of anyone or their families that have been completely destroyed by alcohol abuse? I sure do, including many members of my own family. I have witnessed first-hand the devastation of alcohol addiction and abuse. I could have easily gone down the same path. I CHOSE NOT TO. We all know alcohol can be a horrific drug. Weed, well, not so much. Not even close. Period. I am not suggesting you start using cannabis, but I AM letting you know that it has been extremely beneficial for me as a tool to deal with anxiety and depression with only positive side effects. Once again, I'll state: DON'T LEAVE ANY MONEY ON THE TABLE IN YOUR BATTLE WITH PROSTATE CANCER.

~ ~ ~

Expert Analysis—Dr. Donald Abrams

> My research has been done in the in-patient setting. Cancer patients don't want to spend time that they don't have to in the hospital. I have completed clinical trials in patients with HIV, but most of

my experience is actually anecdotal from being an oncologist for 37 years in San Francisco and seeing so many of my patients benefit from using cannabis.

Ondansetron and Zofran are the two most common anti-nausea prescription medications that we prescribe, and both make people constipated. Cannabis doesn't. If you feel that you're dying, or part of you has died, you really want to be able to continue to move your bowels. That's a big problem that many of my patients have when they get prescribed Ondansetron because they get totally constipated.

The number of patients that I've seen that have been able to wean off of prescription anti-nausea medication and just treat their nausea related to chemo with cannabis is significant.

All cannabis clinical trials to date were done using Delta-9 THC, the main psychoactive component in cannabis. And those trials led to the approval of two different Delta-9 THC formulations in the 1980s for treatment of chemotherapy-induced nausea and vomiting. Dronabinol and Nabilone.

Neither are well tolerated by patients. When you isolate the single most psychoactive component and put it in sesame oil, you remove it basically from the entourage effect that you get from having all of the various cannabinoids as well as the terpenoids and flavonoids present in the plant, which augment the beneficial effects and decrease some of the adverse effects of the Delta-9 THC.

Delta-9 THC takes two-and-a-half hours to reach a peak plasma concentration when eaten. In contrast, when inhaled, the peak plasma concentration is reached in two-and-a-half minutes.

Also, when taken by mouth, cannabis goes through the liver, and the Delta-9 THC gets metabolized into an even more psychoactive 11-hydroxy metabolite. But less of that is formed when the THC is inhaled. That's why people who eat cannabis have an increased psychoactive effect—because more of that 11-hydroxy metabolite is formed than when you inhale it.

If you want that control over the onset, the depth, and the duration of the effect, inhalation is probably better than oral ingestion. There are tinctures and oils that people put under their tongue and swallow. When something is put under the tongue, you get immediate absorption, similar to inhalation, and then when you swallow the rest, you get the same effects as oral ingestion. It's sort of a hybrid kinetics. I recommend tinctures for people that don't want to inhale. Tinctures or oils give you a hybrid of like pharmacokinetics between inhalation and oral ingestion.

We studied the Volcano Vaporizer as a smokeless delivery system in healthy 25 to 40-year-old cannabis smokers and demonstrated that it was as effective as smoking cannabis cigarettes in delivering the chemicals into the bloodstream with less exposure to expired carbon monoxide, which is a marker of exposure to noxious gases in general. (The Volcano is a whole plant vaporizer).

As an oncologist, I tend to be conservative, and I'm all for inhaling plant products, but I've never been comfortable with people inhaling oils. And it seems like that was a wise caution. Don't vape oil. If a patient finds a product that works by mouth for them, and they know how to titrate it, then that's fine. Oils and tinctures that people put under their tongue give you a hybrid kinetics between inhalation and oral ingestion. Some is immediately absorbed from under the tongue, and then oftentimes, you swallow the rest. So that recapitulates the oral ingestion.

The National Cancer Institute has a website (https://www.cancer.gov/about-cancer/treatment/cam/hp/cannabis-pdq), which we update regularly, and it looks at cannabis for symptom management as well as for possible anti-cancer activity. We review all the literature and post it there monthly.

The only studies of cannabis as an anti-cancer agent in humans were done by my friend and colleague, Manuel Guzman, in Spain. His lab studies the effects of cannabinoids on metabolism, and the most metabolically active cells in the body are the brain cells.

Dr. Guzman has done a lot of elegant research demonstrating how cannabinoids directly kill rat brain tumor cells in a test tube. And that has partially led to the enthusiasm that cannabis may have some anti-cancer activity. The highest concentration of the cannabinoid-1 receptors is found in the brain. And so it makes some sense that if you add a cannabinoid, particularly one that might interact with the CB-1 receptor like Delta-9 THC, you may see some effects.

Not only have they demonstrated that cannabis directly kills tumor cells and increases apoptosis, or programmed cell death, but cannabinoids also decrease the vascular endothelial growth factor (VEGF) which promotes new blood vessel formation to feed the tumor so it can grow. They've also demonstrated that cannabinoids depress an enzyme called Matrix Metalloproteinases which allow cancer cells to become invasive and metastasize.

It's all very encouraging, but so far, there's really a paucity of studies in humans. Manuel, who is a PhD and not an MD, went to the Canary Islands and found nine patients who had recurrent glioblastoma multiforme, the most aggressive form of human brain tumor. He dripped Delta-9 THC into their recurrent brain tumor by way of a catheter, and he saw no real difference between those getting chemotherapy alone, compared to those who had the catheter dripping the THC into their brain.

Chapter 17 – Therapy—Cannabis

The next study that was done has not yet been reported in medical literature and is currently only a press release. It's an abstract from the American Society for Clinical Oncology and was a study in patients, again, with recurrent glioblastoma. They had 12 patients use Nabiximol spray under their tongue. Nabiximol is a whole-plant extract that's been modified, so it has a CBD to THC ratio of 1:1. And it's taken as an under-the-tongue spray. It's made by the same company that makes Epidiolex, the CBD product that's been licensed and approved for the treatment of seizures in children.

So, 21 patients with recurrent glioblastoma multiforme are randomized: 12 used the Nabiximol in addition to the chemotherapy and nine sprayed placebos for one year.

At the end of the study, 83% of the group getting Nabiximols were alive compared to 54% of the group getting the placebo. The median survival in the group getting the Nabiximols was 555 days compared to 369 days in the group getting the placebo. But again, the study has not been published yet.

> The biggest question I'm always asked by patients all the time is, "What is the right ratio of THC to CBD that I should take?" My general answer is, "I don't know." But when my brain tumor patients asked me what they should take in conjunction with their temozolomide (chemotherapy), I tell them, "You should do a 1:1 ratio." That's the only information that's available out there at this point.

Two months later, my radiation treatment was done. I received a radiation completion "diploma" from the clinic, and my PSA was undetectable. Great news. My sex drive was also undetectable at this point. I stayed on Lupron and Casodex for one year, and my PSA remained undetectable. It was a reprieve from always seeing my number rise after each blood test for sure, but only time would tell if the radiation had hit the invisible targets in my abdominal lymph nodes. We returned to California and did our best to manage our business, but we were just in a different mind frame at this point. Neither of us wanted to have an office in our house anymore. We let our staff go and downsized or outsourced tasks we did not want to do. I replaced the two desks that our office team had downstairs with a POOL TABLE and stereo, and we bought a hot tub. What a great decision.

I tolerated this round of hormone therapy very easily, and I attribute that primarily to my WFPBD. I maintained my weight, had about the same amount of energy, and I could still surf! Honestly, I was horrified that zeroing out my testosterone would incapacitate my ability to surf. FEAR again was unwarranted in this case. I spent a great deal of time anguishing over my potential loss of manhood, and it was completely unfounded. I was also determined not to let it happen and redoubled my fitness efforts.

Summary

1. Cannabis has the power to safely and gently mitigate the awful side effects of cancer treatment.
2. Due to cannabis' classification as a Schedule 1 narcotic by the federal government, good research is very limited. Don't let any of this stand in your way if cannabis is something you would like to try. It is your decision to make.
3. Being diagnosed with cancer immediately will force you to focus on the truly important things in life—relationships and purpose.

CHAPTER 18
SEX AND INTIMACY

Passionate sex is great. A passionate marriage filled with passionate sex…So much better!

— Anonymous

I love sex. My wife is so HOT. We still cannot keep our hands off of each other after close to 40 years of marriage. My marriage is spectacular. FOCUS on your marriage, not sex.

About two weeks into my first round of HT (hormone therapy), my sex drive was, well, not there. I still felt the need for emotional and physical connection, and I made sure I went out of my way to show Mindy that HT was not going to drive me into an isolationist hole. It's not as if you are really horny, and you can't get it up. It's actually the opposite. I could still get it up; I just wasn't interested in sex. I'd masturbate at least once a week to try to keep blood flow and action going down there, but it was definitely something I forced myself to do. Life is fine without sex if it never enters your mind. HOWEVER, if you are married or have a significant other, I can assure you, their sex drive is still there. It's very easy to forget about this because you are not even thinking of sex, ever. Mindy did a good job of making sure I understood this, and we had sex during hormone therapy. I made sure I satisfied her needs, because, you know, sex is on everyone's mind except those of us on HT.

I need to segue to a very important point here. I am writing this in my RV in a beautiful state park on Lake DeGray in Arkansas in July of 2019. Every doctor we have engaged with on this journey has made the specific point of letting me and Mindy know that, with all of the treatments I have endured, my sexual function is bound to decrease. Specifically, my first radiation oncologist told Mindy that my ability to get and keep an erection would be nil in five years. Utter and complete bullshit. Right now, almost 18 months after completing a 7-month stint on Zytigia along with a second round of Lupron, my sexual function has returned to absolute full capability. Don't believe what you hear. A low-fat, whole-foods, plant-based diet is WAY more powerful than Cialis or Viagra in its ability to restore blood flow to your HEART and your PENIS. It's simply unbelievable. If you are suffering from ED and want to return to sexual glory, EAT A PLANT-BASED DIET! Mindy has written a whole book on this called *The Plant Powered Penis*. Buy it and read it because she outlines the simple truth that, if you want a good erection, a plant-based diet is the best way to do it! The reason why is coming—it's all about creating nitric oxide inside your arteries and veins.

Lesson learned: Go out of your way to display physical love to your partner during HT. Initiate sex even if you don't want it. You don't have to have a raging erection to enjoy intimacy with your loved one. You also now have the ability to focus on YOUR PARTNER'S needs and wants, not yours. This is really important. Ask your wife or significant other what SHE wants! There is no downside to showing your partner how much you love her and pleasing her sexually even if you can't get it up or simply don't care. Take care of your partner's needs—she still has them even if you don't.

Mindy's Perspective

Bruce's doctors were right. Most men do have some form of erectile dysfunction post prostatectomy, radiation, and/or hormone treatment. ED is just accepted as inevitable, so many men relinquish any control that they have to change their outcome. Because I had living proof that the willie doesn't wilt (Bruce's) after treatment, and by doing the research for my book, what we do know is that blood flow to the groin, and for that matter, up the vein chain to the heart and to the head has everything to do with eating a nitric oxide rich diet. And what foods contribute to nitric oxide production in the body? Plant foods: fruits, veggies, grains, beans—all foods created by nature.

As Bruce also mentioned earlier, most doctors don't get an education in nutrition in medical school, so many times their advice to patients is limited to pills and procedures that only mask the symptoms and don't address the underlying problem. It is then our job to support "the system" with all the health-promoting food we can. Make shopping and cooking at home a top priority. Lead by example by fueling your body with health-promoting foods, and if you shop for the family, only purchase food that is supporting great health. If you choose to put something into your cart that is not health-promoting, then what is your message? Be mindful that what you buy will be eaten by someone you love. Do you want to enhance or harm their health? It is that simple.

Summary

1. The side effects of androgen deprivation therapy (ADT) are real, and you must have a strategy to combat them. Exercise and a WFPB diet are powerful tools in dealing with HT.
2. Even if your sex drive has been shot down because of HT, your partner's hasn't.
3. Do everything you can to nurture your relationship through intimacy in all different ways.

CHAPTER 19
WFPB DIET = NO OIL

The fat you eat is the fat you wear.

— Dr. John McDougall

February 13th and 14th, 2016—Another Turning Point—OIL.

Mindy and I attended the McDougall Health Summit in Santa Rosa in 2016. Dr. John McDougall hosts a two-day event a few times every year, where the masterminds of plant-based nutrition convene, lecture, and meet with attendees. During the event, I had the opportunity to meet and talk personally with not only Dr. John McDougall, but also the father of plant-based nutrition, Dr. T. Colin Campbell, Dr. Michael Greger, and Dr. Caldwell Esselstyn. These four pioneers have been on the cutting (and many times bleeding) edge of nutritional science free of pharmaceutical, supplement, or food industry influence.

The event was awesome and inspiring, but even more importantly, Dr. Esselstyn shared his remarkable clinical research on reversing late-stage heart disease with a NO OIL plant-based diet. Additionally, Dr. Greger, Dr. McDougall, and Dr. Esselstyn all shared strong research demonstrating the deleterious effects of consuming so much added FAT in our diets through "free oils," which are isolated manufactured fats that are added to almost ALL processed packaged and restaurant food. "NO OIL!" was the mantra we left with. Stay with me here. It turns out fat, especially saturated fat, impairs cellular oxidation.[1]

Cellular oxidation is what keeps the engines of our cells running in tip-top shape. These "free" fats, including isolated plant fats (canola oil, olive oil, coconut oil, ALL oils), blunt the ability of the endothelial lining in our arteries and veins to deliver nitric oxide into our blood that keeps our arteries flexible and pliable. Dr. Robert Vogel, from the University of Maryland, has demonstrated this process through a series of simple clinical experiments which demonstrate that all fat, even olive oil, slows the ability of our arteries to respond to nitric oxide and dilate.[2]

Bottom line: We have given up eating all oil. All of it, or at least the best we can. It is almost impossible to travel as much as we do, which is basically full time, and avoid all oil. We have developed tactics for finding oil-free food at restaurants, but the best thing you can do is avoid restaurants and cook your meals yourself where you have control of the ingredients, especially oil. Don't be deceived by expensive marketing campaigns claiming

Chapter 19 – WFPB Diet = No Oil

incredible health benefits of consuming unnatural, highly processed 100% fat in the form of free oils. Eliminate the excess fat from your diet, and every cell in your body will thank you! By the way, we have over 30 recipes on video on our website that are completely oil-free. It's all free at onedaytowellness.org.

I'll give you a challenge: Just try to give up added oils and fats to your diet for ONE WEEK. We did, and the contrast is STARK. Now we can taste added oil in any food. It tastes oily and unpleasant. Oil is NOT a healthy food, and you won't be sad you gave it up.

Summary

1. All oils, including plant oils, slow down cellular metabolism, and impair artery function.
2. Try going one week without consuming any added "free" fats to your food.
3. Once you eliminate oil from your diet, you won't want to add it back in.

CHAPTER 20
FINDING MY TEAM

Do not make permanent decisions based off of temporary feelings.

— Brandi Benson

In late June of 2016, within two months of going off HT, my PSA made its appearance known again and began to rise. Crushing. That's the only way I can describe the feeling of hopelessness AGAIN. The year before, we had spent three months in Florida where I was getting radiated every day, taking a boatload of drugs that made me feel sick, and adapting to HT and spending a lot of our own money to do it. And now it seemed like it was a waste of time. Right back where we left off. Rising PSA. This is when I swallowed my pride and called Dr. Scholz at Prostate Oncology Specialists and updated him on what had transpired since our first meeting. I could tell he was NOT HAPPY with my decision to have radiation treatment at the Florida clinic, but he dove right back into my case, and we began to lay out a new plan. He also introduced me to Dr. Jeffrey Turner who is a partner and now my oncologist at PROS.

I felt so relieved and fortunate to be back in this office with this medical team. They didn't shame or blame me for my previous treatment decision. We just started mapping out a new strategy that did not include immediate treatment without knowing where the cancer was. Also, although not nutritional experts, both Dr. Scholz and Dr. Turner understand and acknowledged the importance of diet as an additional adjunct treatment for PC. The team at PROS takes the time to assess the WHOLE individual, not just a specific cancer treatment. Again, I cannot stress the importance of finding the right medical team for your personality and situation. I bumbled and fumbled and let fear drive my decisions up to this point. Did the treatment in Florida help me at all? We will never know for sure, but I can tell you I never felt I connected with that doctor or his clinic. The entire process felt sterile, standoffish, and isolating. This was not the case at PROS. They have a TEAM of oncologists that deal only with PC. Nothing else. The entire staff is well connected to every conceivable medical treatment for PC as well as the best doctors who perform the procedures. The collective team discusses each patient and their progress at weekly meetings to get every doctor's opinion. I trust this team. I trust my personal doctor, who is now Dr. Turner. I have second-guessed every doctor I have engaged with on this PC journey until this point. PROS are my medical oncological generals in my war with PC.

Chapter 20 – Finding My Team

Insurance

By the way, my current insurance, which is now Covered California, does not cover PROS, which really pisses me off. I pay out of pocket for every appointment and probably will until I reach Medicare age, which, as of the writing of this book, is still three years away. Three years seems like a long time while you are watching PSA rise after surgery and radiation and ADT.

Since my last engagement with PROS, the PSMA Ga PET scan had become available at a clinic in Arizona. Dr. Turner wanted me to get this scan before doing anything else. No more throwing darts at an unseen target. He also connected me with Dr. Jeffrey Demanes of UCLA. Dr. Demanes has a stellar reputation for advanced brachytherapy techniques for treating PC and failed RPs. He is also an avid pole vaulter in his late 70s and a really great guy. Both Dr. Turner and Dr. Demanes thought I might still be a candidate for brachytherapy as a curative approach if we could locate the cancer via biopsy and if it was still localized in the prostate bed. We had a plan, and I was feeling emboldened again. Here we go.

Summary

1. Take the time (and money if necessary) to look outside of your insurance network for expert medical guidance on PC. Slow down.
2. If you are not comfortable being completely open with your medical team, you need to keep looking.

3. Reach out to one of the many PC specialists listed in the resource section of this book.

CHAPTER 21
FIND YOUR PURPOSE

It's not enough to have lived. We should be determined to live for something.

— Winston Churchill

October 15th, 2016—We Launch One Day to Wellness

While all of this PC crap was ongoing for me, Mindy and I decided to launch our new nutritional educational program, One Day to Wellness. Fitness pros need to maintain their continuing education credits just like nurses and dietitians. This is usually accomplished through a dizzying selection of certifications offered by accredited fitness councils such as ACE (American Council on Exercise) and AFPA (American Federation of Professional Athletes). There is literally NO one-day certification on plant-based nutrition in the fitness industry, and we decided to put one together.

It was a massive undertaking, but Mindy is an excellent organizer and planner. We broke up the project into parts and architected what is now the ONLY 9-hour plant-based nutrition certification available in the fitness industry.

It is an AWESOME, life-changing day. Not only do we cover the science and research, but we also spend time helping participants understand behavioral change strategies that have worked for us, mindfulness, nutritional programming, and the critical importance of moving your body throughout the day.

Since our first certification in October of 2016, we have provided this live, nine-hour certification, over 100 times with over 2000 people completing it and still counting. We have added a second day to One Day to Wellness called "Cooking and Coaching," where we teach people how to cook delicious plant-based food.

I love it all. Nutritional science has become my passion and my PURPOSE over the last nine years. I LOVE nutritional science. Diving into this world has been a god-send for me in dealing with cancer. My sense of purpose drives me to continue my education; it motivates me to drive my engagement with hundreds of people who are HUNGRY to improve their health, and it keeps me very BUSY. I have NEVER been more satisfied with work than I am right now. Some people never truly figure out what their passion and mission in life are, but I am fortunate enough to be someone who has.

Take action! NOW is the time to do what you want to do. Figure out what you really love to do and do it.

Chapter 21 – Find Your Purpose

Having a purpose will help you in your cancer battle as well as the rest of your life. It doesn't have to be complicated, but you need a good reason to wake up in the morning other than slogging through another day in a job you don't like (I spent many years in this situation and looking back, I should have made a big change much sooner than I did). Don't let FEAR stand in your way of making drastic changes in your life as well as your diet! Take that first step. It took me over 50 years to figure it out.

Summary

1. Find your purpose and dive in.
2. Never stop learning.
3. Don't let fear hold you back from living the life you imagined.

CHAPTER 22
ITALY AND FASTING

Adding something, and therefore "doing something," seems much more intuitively reasonable than subtracting the "unlikely" causes and letting the body heal itself.

— Dr. Douglas J. Lisle

Italy trip - March 2017

Drop everything you are doing and book a 10-day self-guided bike tour through Tuscany. Do it now! What an incredible trip. Riding for 20 to 30 miles every day and ending up at a different mountain town every night WITH ALL OF YOUR STUFF WAITING FOR YOU in your quaint historic hotel!

NOW is the time to start doing all the stuff you always said you were going to do, but work and life always got in the way. During this 10-day pedal through the wine country of Italy, I brought the book, *The Pleasure Trap*, by Dr. Alan Goldhamer and Dr. Douglas

Lisle. Buy the book. You can read it in two hours. It might change your life.

The biking was epic; the book was life-altering. Drs. Lisle and Goldhamer outline in *The Pleasure Trap* their work at the medically supervised fasting clinic, The TrueNorth Health Center in Santa Rosa, CA. What's going on there? Just reversing diabetes, lupus, arthritis, heart disease, AND SLOWING AND EVEN REVERSING THE GROWTH OF SOME CANCERS, including prostate, breast, and blood cancers. How do they do it? They show you how to stop eating first. Patients at TrueNorth are clinically supervised and water-only fast anywhere from just a few days to up to 40 days. Water only. What happens? People with lifelong chronic diseases, on scores of medications, simply get better because the major injury to their bodies (consuming too many animal products and processed foods) is removed. Remarkably simple and more effective than any drug available.

I was intrigued by this concept of fasting to regain health and wanted to give it a try. It turns out that fasting benefits every cell in your body through a process called autophagy which is the body's way of cleaning out damaged cells, in order to regenerate newer, healthier ones. "Auto" means self, and "phagy" means eat. So, the literal meaning of autophagy is "self-eating." Autophagy only happens after all of the glucose is used up in your body, which can take up to three days of water-only fasting. After that, the magic of autophagy begins when

Chapter 22 – Italy and Fasting

your body shifts the metabolic pathway of burning the body's preferred fuel, glucose, to burning fat for energy.

The book and the research blew me away. It would be another year before I finally got the guts to commit to actually checking myself and Mindy into TrueNorth and DOING IT, but I was going to DO IT. I just needed to find the window in our schedule which turned out to be almost 18 months later, which I'll discuss in an upcoming section.

Summary

1. Pull out that "bucket list" and get started NOW!
2. Buy the book, *The Pleasure Trap*, and read it.
3. Fasting is HARD but worth it.

CHAPTER 23
BUT FIRST MORE TESTS

Medical science is making such remarkable progress that soon none of us will be well.

— ALDOUS HUXLEY

But first! April 2017 Ga PET (gallium PET scan) in Arizona. PSA was at 0.60, well within the range of the Ga PET scan's ability to detect cancer. The scan in Arizona showed a possible, but not confirmed, hot spot in my lower left prostate bed. The lower left area of what is now just a place where my prostate used to be is where my positive margin was located prior to prostate removal. Everything pointed to the lower left. OK. Next up: Biopsy at UCLA in the summer of 2017 is scheduled. Our business is the most busy and hectic in the summer, and Mindy and I are traveling nonstop on airplanes crossing the country. The only available appointment for the biopsy at UCLA was in August, one week prior to the largest fitness conference in North America: CanFitPro in Toronto. I was also informed by a good friend that it was really important that Mindy and

I attend the opening ceremonies of the event because we were going to be the recipients of their LifeTime Achievement award for that year. Really? Me? Mindy, of course. She's a legend. I am just a recent appearance as a lecturer and presenter in this world. Apparently, our commitment to delivering the truth about evidence-based nutrition without corporate sponsorship was getting noticed. I was NOT going to miss this ceremony. The last award I can remember getting was for the 50-meter free style in junior high! We scheduled the biopsy at UCLA medical center two days before the award event in Toronto.

And the biopsy was... negative. If we can't see it, we can't go in and get it. Now what?

Prior to this biopsy, Mindy and I met again in the summer of 2017 with Dr. Turner. The new drug, Zytiga, was just approved for non-metastatic, non-hormone refractory PC, and Dr. Turner was excited to give us this news. We agreed I would do a seven-month course of Zytiga with Lupron. I began in June of 2017 and finished at the end of December 2017. How was it? Well, pretty easy as far as handling the side effects. Dr. T. had warned me of the potential potent side effects (read: effects) of the drug combo. Tired, feeling bloated, no sex drive, weight gain, nausea, and on and on. It was a breeze for me. Yes, my sex drive disappeared again, but as you now know, I didn't care! With the exception of zeroing out the horniness factor, I felt, well, great. It was also a tremendous boost to my psyche and Mindy's because, once again, my PSA dropped to undetectable.

Chapter 23 – But First More Tests

Dr. T was quite surprised and pleased with how I handled the treatment. Once again, I have to let you know, it is my DIET that is my most powerful tool in minimizing treatment side effects. Yes, I am younger than most men who have to start to deal with this, but my ability to handle these caustic treatments is because I am fueling my body the way it wants.

Be Prepared

It is very important for me to have questions ready prior to a doctor's meeting. Having my support team there with me assures me that I won't miss anything as well. I also express my emotional and mental concerns. Just remember, your doc is there to help, but he or she needs feedback from us to determine how best to proceed on the medical front.

Here is an example of an email communication prior to my visit:

> Hello Dr. Turner:
>
> I REALLY wanted to meet with you at your office on Friday, but we won't be able to get to Santa Monica by then. Still hoping there might be a cancellation on your schedule Monday, Tuesday, or Wednesday of next week, but if not, let's plan on a phone conference on Friday at 2:30 p.m. instead of an office visit.

I finally mustered up the courage to read *The Key to Prostate Cancer: 30 Experts Explain 15 Stages of Prostate Cancer.* I read the entire book two days ago. Great book, including the chapter on "Health Issues." But of course, it scares me. Of all of the classifications outlined, I did not see any reference to T3b pathology after surgery. I am still not sure where I am on the blue scale. Based on my history, I think I am high Azure, but I am not yet hormone-refractory. (To provide you with some clarity, the book categorizes the stages of cancer by hews of the color blue. The darker the color, the fewer the options.)

What is my PSA doubling time?

Because of our travel schedule, I have been having my PSA done by Quest. The test before this most recent one six weeks ago was 1.1, but I don't think it was ultra-sensitive, just regular PSA. Does this make a difference in determining doubling time? I have read that there can be as much as a 20% difference between the regular and ultra-sensitive. Is that true?

Based on our current situation, do you think my window of potential cure is closed or closing? Based on that answer,

> should I continue to do nothing and monitor PSA? If so, what is the target and cut off for going back on hormones?
>
> Should we schedule another PSMA scan and possible biopsy again?
>
> Do you think the immediate PSA relapse post TIP is indicative of metastatic disease even though we have not been able to locate via biopsy?
>
> If I go back on just bicalutamide, do you think it will suppress the cancer again and make it more difficult to locate, delaying a potential curative approach?

Dr. Scholz's book cites very compelling research on long-term statin use being correlated with reduced metastatic disease. My cholesterol hovers between 185 and 190 on a strict plant-based, low-fat diet. I've got the statins in my medicine cabinet (along with bicalutamide) but have yet to implement.

> Do you think I should begin a long-term statin regime?
>
> Same goes for low dose aspirin. Does recent research suggest the risks outweigh the potential benefits?
>
> I know you already know this, but I am having difficulty emotionally right now. The state of complete limbo is taxing.

> Again, physically, I feel fantastic. I am in better shape than I have ever been, even in my 20s! Up until this last PSA, my mental and emotional outlook has been generally positive, but this one hit me hard. I am still determined to do whatever I have to do. You and your team are my generals in this battle. I believe I have the best generals there are.

These questions give ME a guideline when having a meeting with my doctor when I know my emotions and state of mind are fragile and on guard. I also hope it gives Dr. T some insight into not just my physical state, but my emotional frame of mind. Take the time to write down the major concerns you have with your doctor and get it to them in an email before your visit. It will help both you and your doctor.

So, the biopsy at UCLA showed no sign of cancer. Nothing. Great! Not Great?! Now what? Although my PSA had dropped to zero with the HT/Zytigia treatment, I knew through previous experience that my nadir (lowest measurement) PSA of zero would probably not last after completing the medication course, but Dr. Turner and I still had hope that the Zytigia might help slow things down. Well, within two months of ending the treatment in December of 2017, my PSA started to rise AGAIN. At this point, my brain does feel like it's about to explode. Meditation is helping but, COME ON MAN—

yet another whack from the blood lab showing in a pretty graph my PSA acceleration. Dr. Turner and I both hoped for a longer-term remission after completion of Zytigia, but it just didn't happen.

Mindy's Perspective

Go to every appointment with him. He needs you now more than ever to be the shoulder to lean on and their second set of ears because theirs don't work so well during these appointments. You are there to remember to ask the pertinent questions and to bring up sensitive issues that he may not bring up on his own. Take notes and know the details so that you are sitting at the table well educated and as an equal team member.

Summary

1. Write down your questions prior to your appointment and email it to your doctor at least one day prior to your meeting. Preparation on your part will be appreciated and respected by your medical team.
2. Educate yourself on your stage and treatment options as best you can prior to an appointment.
3. Always take your caregiver with you to your doctor's appointment.

CHAPTER 24
BREAKFAST WITH DR. GREGER AT IDEA IN JULY 2017 AND THE WELLNESS WAGON

> *Successful people are always looking for opportunities to help others. Unsuccessful people are always asking, "What's in it for me?"*
>
> — Brian Tracy

Life goes on despite cancer battles. IDEA is the largest health and fitness conference in the US and takes place every July. This year, Dr. Michael Greger of Nutritionfacts.org was speaking at their nutrition and wellness track. Mindy and I had breakfast with Dr. G before his lecture, which was the catalyst for us to form our foundation, One Day to Wellness.

Mindy and I had met Dr. Greger a year earlier for a video—a taped interview which you can watch on our website (https://onedaytowellness.org/interviews/). He loved our passion and that we had created the One Day to Wellness (ODTW) program. He agreed to lend us his support as an educational sponsor as well as review some of my presentations on plant-based science with one caveat: We had to become a 501(c)3 non-profit and agree not to take any sponsorship money from the food, drug, or supplement industry. He firmly believes, as do I, that as soon as an organization, non-profit or not, begins to accept money from industry sponsors, their message is going to become skewed towards their sponsor's position. It happens all the time. We agreed during that breakfast and launched our non-profit OneDayToWellness.org that summer.

Later that summer, Mindy and I were flying back and forth and up and down all over North America presenting our ODTW program at fitness clubs, YMCA's, and community centers as well as presenting at every single fitness conference available. There are a lot of them. In a typical year, we will be on the schedule at 20+ conferences in Canada and the US. It's incredibly satisfying work; we both love it, but we were literally living in airports, airplanes, car rental counters, and hotels. I was fed up with all of the air travel. I remember sitting on a bench at some mall in Atlanta, GA, about to go to the airport to fly back to San Francisco, drive the hour to our house in Santa Cruz, catch up on office work for ONE DAY and then drive back to SF airport, fly to DC, and start the cycle all over again—while also trying to manage the stress and anxiety of a PC life.

What am I DOING TO MYSELF? I HATE airplane travel. I put my foot down. I told Mindy that she was welcome to fly across the country and return two

Chapter 24 – Breakfast with Dr. Greger at IDEA...

days later to DC, but I WAS NOT GETTING ON AN AIRPLANE. We had no need to return to California. Our home office was GONE (thank you!), and our kids were all adults living their own lives. No dog. No cat. The plants can fend for themselves. I told Mindy I was going to stay in Atlanta an extra day at the hotel, RELAX, and then rent a car and drive the six or so hours to Washington, DC. No airports. Min put up a bit of a protest, something along the lines of "but we need to do laundry," but she eventually came to the realization that I WAS RIGHT. If we were going to keep up this work schedule, it could not include an airport every other day.

Lightbulb Moment #1: I always admired the way John Madden managed to attend and broadcast an endless amount of football games all over the country and never step foot in an airplane. He was definitely on to something. "Mindy, we are going to buy an RV and become the John and Jane Madden of nutrition and wellness!" Just one problem: I am pretty sure John Madden makes more money than we do. There's just not a lot of money in explaining to people they need to eat more fruits, veggies, and grains. But I was not going to be deterred. We went to an RV sales showroom as soon as we got back to CA from DC.

Long story short: We bought a used 2008 Itasca Winnebago during Thanksgiving week of 2017 with 6k miles on it and in perfect condition at a ridiculously great price. And we immediately put it in storage. We had to lay out our travel schedule for 2018. We also had to figure out how we would PAY for this non-profit traveling RV mission. Our business was still generating income, and we were beginning to make money as lecturers and educators, but it wasn't 1990s Silicon Valley high tech sales type of money. I didn't care. We committed to one year of traveling in the RV. We decided to rent out our beautiful, newly remodeled beach house in Santa Cruz. And we found the perfect family as renters, and they are still living in our home today. The rental income of our beach house allowed us to take the leap into full-time RV road living which also continues to this day. (Thank you Harmon's!)

Lightbulb Moment #2: The WRAP! Mindy's brother, an avid RV'er, had plenty of suggestions, but the best one was "you should wrap the whole RV in your logo and fruits and vegetables." We already had a burgeoning business selling fruit and veggie tee shirts at events, and this would be the perfect branding extension. YES, PLEASE. We drove the RV from Santa Cruz to have the RV wrapped in our signature fruit and veggie theme along with our broccoli One Day to Wellness logo. Best idea ever. We now travel full time in the RV which also acts as our billboard on the road and our booth at larger trade shows and conventions. It stands out, which is perfect. We have learned that being a scientifically evidenced-based health educator and advocate is a little like being a vampire. YOU NEED AN INVITATION TO COME IN! We NEVER reach out or discuss our non-profit mission with anyone, unless they ask. The fruit

Chapter 24 – Breakfast with Dr. Greger at IDEA...

and veggie wrapped RV encourages people to ask: "What in the hell are you guys doing?" THAT is the invitation. From there, we simply say, "We are a non-profit organization, and we help people understand evidenced-based nutrition. Here is a flyer with some information and a list of our educational partners. If you have any questions, we would be more than happy to discuss it with you." That's it. No, "Don't eat animals." No, "I'm a vegan and you should be too!" Just a smile and a piece of non-threatening literature. People always want to know more. The door always opens up.

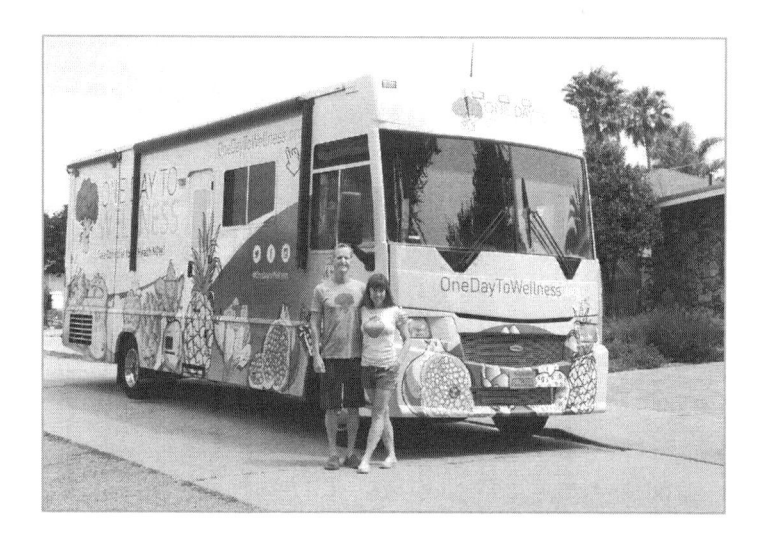

We left on our virgin voyage from Santa Cruz in February of 2017 and have NEVER looked back. If we knew how much fun it would be to live and work from an RV, we would have done it 10 years sooner. It's awesome. I am writing this section of the book in bed in the back of the RV at a stunningly beautiful state park on Lake DeGray in Arkansas. It cost $8 a night. We are here for a week. I plan on finishing the book right here. (I didn't.)

Anyway, in the spring of 2017, the PSMA scan was approved by the FDA as an advanced diagnostic tool for recurrent, non-metastatic PC. The current PSA cut off to be accepted for the PSMA scan was 0.035. By June of 2018 my PSA was already at 0.417 and rising at this point, so I was qualified. Lucky me.

My first PSMA scan was at UCLA on July 3rd, 2018. At this point, only UCLA and UCSF had the equipment and trained staff to perform the procedure. We chose UCLA because we were now living in the RV full time, and we were visiting our two older boys who both lived in LA. The PSMA scan revealed (again) a potential hot-spot in the lower-left base of my prostate bed. Deja Vu. Armed with this new potential cancer site as a target, Dr. Turner and PROS arranged my second post RP biopsy a week later. We were in transit as usual, this time staying at our lifelong friends.

Side Note: Know your closest friends and make sure you nurture those relationships as if they were a top priority in your life. They usually are. I met my best friend, Jeff Llewellyn, my first week as a freshman at the University of Florida back in 1980. We connected, lived together on and off in college, along with Chris who is now Jeff's wife. Jeff is the only person, other than Mindy, that I feel comfortable sharing ALL of my feelings and emotions with. He's the brother I never had. I try to be completely honest with my three boys about my mental struggles in dealing with the disease, but innately, I also keep a stiff upper lip with them because I just don't want to bring them down.

In one day, we parked the RV at Jeff and Chris' house, borrowed their car, drove to the airport, flew to LA, completed the biopsy procedure, and flew back to Denver that night. It was an exhausting couple of days, and I was in a fair amount of pain post-biopsy. Two days later, we get the report back from LA: Biopsy……. NEGATIVE…. again. No cancer detected. Great!! Horrible!! Why is my PSA going up, and we can't find cancer anywhere? At this point, I have completely recovered from the Zytiga/Lupron protocol I was on for seven months. I was, as usual, feeling physically spectacular. Plenty of energy, no pain, daily full erections, surfing a lot, and now 60 years old with the dark shadow of cancer following me around everywhere I go.

Summary

1. NOW is the time to take stock in your life and how you live.
2. Take more risks.
3. Don't ever give up.

CHAPTER 25
TRUENORTH FASTING ADVENTURE SEPTEMBER 2018

I fast for greater physical and mental efficiency.

— Plato

I was willing to try just about anything at this point with my rising PSA. As you may recall, I had scheduled an intake meeting at TrueNorth Fasting Clinic in the early summer of 2018 where I also did a video interview with the founder, Dr. Alan Goldhamer. You can watch the interview on our website, onedaytowellness.org. We also met with several of the medical staff at the facility. Based on our consultation, we agreed that I would attempt an 11-day, water-only fast, and Mindy would attempt an 8-day, water-only fast during the late summer of 2018 at TNHC. Why Mindy? We both wanted first-hand research on this very hot topic if we were going to speak about fasting. And research demonstrates, clearly, there is only a health upside to extended water-only fasting.

My PSA was 0.63 the week before we checked in. We followed the "down feeding" procedure outlined by Dr. Goldhamer, which consists of cutting back on solid food for the four days prior to the fast with the day before being juice only.

We were ready to go when we arrived at the TrueNorth Health Center (TNHC). Go where? Do what? I guess I'll wait for lunch....... oh..... there is no lunch. There is plenty of water! TNHC does a great job of keeping you busy and providing both live and recorded educational content on why you are doing what you are doing. There are usually two or three lectures each day by one of the attending physicians on staff covering the science of fasting and its power to bring the body back to homeostasis very quickly. Water only fasting is EXTREMELY powerful and fast acting. Here is the thing. I checked into TrueNorth weighing in at 133 pounds. I am 5'10". If you do the BMI (Body Mass Index) calculation, this puts me at the lower end of the healthy BMI scale, exactly where experts want it to be. Go Bruce. However, most people checking into TrueNorth are there to bring themselves back from metabolic catastrophes such as diabetes, angina, heart disease, or arthritis. Typically, these issues (just like PC) come along with excess weight. When water-only fasting, after two or three days, your body has utilized whatever glucose is left in your body tract for fuel. Once all this fuel is used up, our bodies then begin accessing glycogen from our muscle tissues and our liver. Once THAT fuel is used up, the body begins to enter a state of ketosis, which I am sure you have heard about. The body begins producing ketones from fat stores as the fuel source for the brain, and the only reserves left in the body are….. FAT. So fat begins to be consumed.

If you arrive at TrueNorth and begin a water-only fast with a lot of fat on your frame, your body begins the process of burning up all that fat, and hunger is suppressed, making it easier not to eat. If you have very few or NO lipid reserves (Bruce and Mindy), you very quickly go into ketosis, and you need to be monitored by a doctor very closely. I was hungry the whole time I was there! Both Mindy's and my lower back hurt, especially at night. This is very common with water-only fasting and is attributed to your kidneys going into overdrive filtration, processing the metabolic change that is happening to your body along with their job of clearing toxins from your tissues. How much am I paying to be miserable every day? Also, sleep was not easy. Back pain, hunger, and no A/C at the facility in the inland Central California heat made it difficult to sleep for an extended period. But I was pumped, psyched, and motivated to push through all of it and see if I could slow down my PSA velocity. Dr. Goldhamer and I had no expectations that we would see a serious change or remission, but we both hoped for the best. Additionally, Dr. G. had documented several case studies of certain cancers, such as Stage 3 lymphoma, going into complete remission at his clinic.[1]

And there we were. We had a TV in our room. I was hungry. I was not eating. I decided to do a marathon binge and watch every cooking show imaginable. Anthony Bourdain, Andrew Zimmer, Guy Fieri. Mindy thought I was crazy. I thought I was living vicariously through food shows. We were counseled to expect our hunger to diminish on the second or third day of the fast. I was hungry all the time.

Mindy was not going to make it to seven days, and I was not going to make it to eleven days. At the end of Mindy's fifth day of WOF (water-only fasting), she went back on juice. She went from 112 to 98 pounds in five days and had ZERO energy.

I soldiered on for a total of eight days of WOF. I was determined to continue, but I could barely stand up and walk. My doctor checked my pulse at the end of the eighth day while I was lying on a lounge chair dreaming of tacos. I had gone from 133 pounds to 121 pounds in eight days. This was definitely at the threshold of starvation. He said, "Bruce, you have NO pulse. You are ending your fast today. We are going to start you on diluted celery and watermelon juice right now!" I was THRILLED. The staff brought me the juice. The first sip of this diluted juice and water tasted sweeter and more delicious than anything I had ever ingested in my entire life. My taste buds had completely recalibrated themselves to baseline again. When this happens, EVERYTHING tastes incredibly salty and delicious.

Chapter 25 – TrueNorth Fasting Adventure...

The refeeding process was the down-feeding process in reverse. A day of juice, then simple solids, then, back to a whole-food plant-based low-fat, SOS free (no added salt, oil, or sugar) diet.

Here is the thing: After completing this fast, my energy level, attitude, and mood in general, shot through the roof. It was as if I had been injected with water from the fountain of youth. My skin looked amazing. I looked amazing. I FELT amazing; my blood pressure was perfect; my triglycerides were perfect. WOW! I was, and still am, sold on water-only fasting. The staff was adamant that I wait at least four weeks before checking my PSA to let my whole system calm down, and I reluctantly agreed. (Who's an expert on waiting for blood tests? ME).

At the end of the fasting protocol at TrueNorth, Dr. Goldhamer has only one prescription for ALL of his patients: Going forward, eat only a whole-food, low-fat, SOS free (no added salt, oil, or sugar) diet, and schedule an appointment to come back for a checkup in 50 YEARS. Meaning, if you can stay on the WFPB with no SOS diet, in all likelihood, your metabolic symptoms will NEVER come back. This should give everybody a good indication of what the problem was that got them to the point of having to starve themselves back to homeostasis. It's the food. It's always been the food, and it will always be the food. Fix the food, and most everything will take care of itself. No calculators, no calorie counting, no limiting portions. Don't eat what we now know are disease-promoting foods. Eat health-promoting foods, and your body will heal itself. Don't bother even considering water-only fasting if your plan is to go back to eating the SAD (Standard American Diet) of ultra-processed foods and animal products. Is it easy? No. Nothing is easy in a cancer battle. Not mine.

DON'T LEAVE ANY MONEY ON THE TABLE IN YOUR CANCER BATTLE.

Summary

1. Medically supervised water-only fasting has been proven to slow or reverse the growth of many forms of cancer, although there is little data available for PC.
2. Fasting is the most powerful tool available to reset your metabolism.
3. Reach out to TrueNorth! They want to help.

CHAPTER 26
BREAKDOWN #2

We get anxious more with imaginations than actuality.

— Abhijit Naskar

The breakdown: the triggers, then the flood of uncontrollable emotions. And here's how it happens. We are in Colorado and have spent four wonderful days in Denver with Jeff and Chris. I am at a crossroads AGAIN with PC. Seven and a half years after initial diagnosis: My PSA has been rising since coming off of a six-month plan of Zytiga + Lupron almost 17 months ago. Six weeks ago, it was 1.1, and I just got the results from my test three days ago from Quest: 1.37. Just when I thought it might be slowing down, the gut-punch hits me again. I should be completely numb from almost eight years of blood tests, but the truth is, it's always anguishing waiting for the results and still devastating when it's not good. What am I expecting? I know it's not going DOWN! I received the results from Dr. Turner's office while in Jeff and Chris's living room, and it was crushing. Thank God I was with people who truly cared for me. I had two glasses of rum, and we all talked it out in their living room. The four of us hugged. As previously stated, I can't emphasize how important it is to have people close enough to you to be able to let yourself go emotionally with them during the dark moments. Mindy is always there as my first line of defense, but having my closest friends there was a bonus.

Also, our RV slide-out broke AGAIN and was being worked on AGAIN at a local RV repair shop just outside of Denver. It was now functional $2000 later. Every repair on an RV is $2000 minimum in our experience. But we need the space the slide-out provides because we LIVE in it. That extra three feet of width means a lot, and it was finally working again! We said goodbye to Denver and began our journey west to Anaheim for the IDEA World Fitness Conference where the RV will be on the trade show floor.

While we were waiting for the RV to get repaired, Mindy and I rode our bikes to downtown Denver for the day to kill time. As part of the research for this book, I had purchased a book by Dr. Mark Scholz of PROS, *The Key to Prostate Cancer*. It's an excellent book and very well researched. Buy it and read it. The truth is I have had the book for over a year, but I was afraid to open it. I hid from it. I was afraid to read it because I did not want to know my "stage of blue." (Instead of identifying cancer as low, medium, high risk, relapsing, or metastatic diseases, Dr. Scholz uses different shades of "blue" for identifying cancer.)

Chapter 26 – Breakdown #2

But I had Dr. Scholz's book with me, and I read it cover to cover that day in Denver. It's a book of hope, but it confirmed what I have always known: My situation is classified as high risk, to say the least. The book outlines the 12 stages of prostate cancer, and each stage is identified as a hue of blue color. "Sky" is the first sage of blue, then "Teal," then "Azure," then "Indigo," and finally, two stages of "Royal." I'm "Early Royal," the LAST, darkest color of blue. Early Royal translates to "limited options." In addition, I just got the blood test back the day before that confirmed my PSA's continual rise. Getting gut-punched with another rising PSA while reading and doing a deep dive into PC research is a fine balancing act. I wanted to keep my head in the sand as long as possible, but I know I need to arm myself with research to make the best treatment decisions. I don't like what the research says about my condition. I hate it actually. It's going to depress me, but I am compelled to deal with it. DEAL with it. Face your fears and accept them. I'm a work in progress, but I AM doing better.

Okay. RV repaired, and we are now on our way to California. We said goodbye to Denver and our friends and began our journey west to Anaheim for the IDEA World Fitness Conference where the RV will be on the trade show floor.

After a few hours of driving, we pull into a really nice campground. We deploy the slide and…… it locks up again! It doesn't go out. It's 9 p.m., and it's raining. I lose it. I smash my fist into the counter top, and then the now-familiar uncontrollable flood of emotions begins to pour over me. I can't see a way out. My mental capacity shuts down. I can feel the cracks opening up on my mental stability. I cry it out, again, with Mindy. Thank God for Mindy. I hate the situation, I hate myself for breaking down, I hate the fact that I know how much it hurts the ones closest to me to see me go through this. And it is worse—I am lost, depressed, and I see no way out. I hate THAT. It hurt's so bad I taste it, and it feels like it's never going to end. It's simply awful. I let it all go with Mindy that night. If I did not have the emotional support from my dearest friends and family, I don't think I could survive this journey.

The depression passes the next day. It always does. REMEMBER THAT: As horrible as the situation may seem, it will pass. There will be a better day.

The next day, we troubleshoot the slide-out situation on the phone with the RV tech in Denver and fixed it again! We camped in Palisade, Colorado, which is stunningly beautiful. The slide-out works. I know I have a phone meeting with Dr. Turner tomorrow. I trust him. I trust my friends. I trust my family. I will move forward. Keep moving forward. I don't want to have any more mental breakdowns, but I know I probably will. I call it a breakdown, but what it really is, is the learned skill of being able to completely let go emotionally with the people that I care about most. I am crying as I write this. Let it go. Let it go with the people you love. Drop the facade, the macho bullshit, the tough veneer. Let it all go. You will be a better person. You will be better able to cope. It will make you a better MAN. It did for me!

Summary

1. Just like RVs, people break down.
2. Give yourself permission to be emotional and vulnerable. You deserve it.
3. Take the time to process and contemplate what leads up to an emotional crisis.

CHAPTER 27
I CHOSE TO BE HAPPY

*Let your tears flow and where they go,
let your sorrows follow.*

— Dodinsky

Today, we are riding our bikes to downtown Palisade. It's beautiful here. The weather is perfect. I am going to have a good day. The emotional pain subsides. Remember that. At its darkest moment, the emotional pain seems insurmountable, but it doesn't last. Don't let it take you down. Learn how to use the tools available to you to MANAGE the pain and communicate to someone you trust what is happening to you.

At this point, almost nine years after initial diagnosis, one RP, at least 40 blood tests, two bone scans, three CAT scans, two MRI's, three biopsies, and two PSMA scans, all unable to definitively locate cancer, I have become a full-on, full-time cancer warrior. I feel EMPOWERED and in control of my health. I am empowered by the challenge and discipline of water-only fasting. I am empowered by my ability to change my lifelong diet of GARBAGE to eating health-promoting foods. (It's all I want to eat now, which is a testament that if I can go from a lifelong diet of the worst possible food for your health to only eating foods that improve my health, ANYONE can do it!)

YOU can do this, and you should, because chances are you are trying to save your life. I stopped feeding my cancer, and so can you. Reach out! I'm here to help, and so are a growing cadre of well-meaning organizations such as Physician's Committee for Responsible Medicine (https://www.pcrm.org/),
Nutritionfacts.org
(https://nutritionfacts.org/video/survival-of-the-firmest-erectile-dysfunction-and-death/)
and Foodrevolution.org (https://foodrevolution.org/), just to name a few.

I'd like to say that getting blood tests is becoming easier, but I'd be lying. Maybe they are becoming slightly less anxiety-ridden, but the wait to get the results is still TOUGH. And even though I know and expect my PSA to keep going up, it's still a gut punch when I see the upward trend of the graph. I would describe it as "becoming better at managing my emotions, and I know the feeling of hopelessness and fear will mitigate over the next 24 hours, and I'll be that much more at peace."

Dr. Turner and I have been monitoring my PSA very closely since going off the Zytiga at the end of 2018. Just over two years later, and my PSA, as of two weeks ago is 2.63.

Chapter 27 – I Chose to be Happy

We will continue to monitor for the time being as my doubling time seems to have slowed down to about 10 months since my water-only fasting treatment at TrueNorth. Our current plan is to probably do another PSMA scan/biopsy next month. Dr. T wants me to do a blood test every month. I am going to go every eight weeks.

So here I sit in our "Wellness Wagon" RV. Physically, I feel better than I have in my entire life. Mentally, I have learned to utilize the tools of mindfulness and meditation to manage the fear and anxiety that I will always have. I have completely turned my diet around, bringing my cholesterol, blood pressure, triglycerides, and C-reactive protein to very healthy levels. I have found my true passion in life (better late than never): Helping others understand the power of evidence-based nutrition and helping them improve their lives. My wife and I live full time in a fruit and veggie covered RV, and we are happier than we have ever been. I have three wonderful sons that love me and would do anything for me (I would do anything for them). I have a select few (you don't need many) lifelong friends that would do anything for me, and I would do anything for them.

My cancer is still there somewhere and growing, but I am doing everything I can to keep it at bay. Do I still freak out and have an emotional letdown when my PSA goes up, the slide breaks again on my RV, and I'm stranded in the rain? Yes, and it feels GOOD when it's over! I have expanded my toolbox of techniques to deal with the MENTAL weight of my whole situation. It's still tough, but I am getting better at it every day. Since diagnosis, and since adopting a WFPBD-SOS free diet, I have never felt sick except when I was on the prescription drugs during my Florida radiation treatment. I simply never get sick anymore like I used to several times a year when eating the SAD.

Through nine years of bumbling and fear-induced decisions, actions, and reactions, I have finally found the medical team that I trust and am comfortable with. And from a career perspective, I am the most satisfied and fulfilled that I have ever been in my life. If there is a gift from PC, this is it. Cancer forced me to face my demons, forced me to face my destructive behaviors, forced me to develop mental and physical tools to cope with life's fears and anxieties (which we all have), forced me to be patient and thorough in selecting a medical team, and most importantly it forced me to LEARN HOW TO MAKE DRASTIC CHANGES IN MY BEHAVIOR (all for the better) that I otherwise would have never considered.

I may not have wiped out my cancer, but I have learned to live with it and to make every day I DO HAVE on this planet the best that I can. Cancer has made me a better person. Crazy. If this easily addicted, old surf-bum from Santa Cruz can turn his life around after a cancer diagnosis at 52, SO CAN YOU! WHAT'S THE DOWNSIDE?

Chapter 27 – I Chose to be Happy

Mindy's Perspective

Bruce is a different man today than nine years ago. Precancer Bruce would deal in the "It's-all-good" space. If everything was running smoothly, then all was good. No huge highs and no deep lows—just status quo is how Bruce liked it. Post cancer Bruce has huge highs and a few deep lows. This way of living is better, in my opinion. Don't get me wrong. I am in no way saying that cancer is a good thing. However, knowing that life is finite means Bruce doesn't take anything for granted, and he wants to live—really live, not just exist. So many of us go through life just crossing things off our To-Do lists. We plan a path and then follow it. We don't often veer. Well, Bruce has veered, and it is good because he is rich in emotion, gratitude, and selflessness.

Summary

1. You are responsible for your health. You make the decisions.
2. Choose to be happy and to live every day in a meaningful way.
3. A cancer diagnosis CAN make you a better person if you let it.

PART 2

CHAPTER 28
DIGGING DEEPER

It is never too late to be who you might have been.

— George Eliot

No one wants to believe they caused their own cancer, me included. However, a systematic review of the research to date leaves no question in my mind: I brought my own cancer on and continued to fuel its growth by eating a diet dominated by meat, dairy, eggs, and high fat processed foods for 53 years. According to the American Cancer Institute, research has shown that a poor diet and not being active are two key factors that can increase a person's cancer risk.[1]

I personally do not feel shame or blame myself or anyone else for this outcome. We simply did not have the breadth and depth of population, epidemiological, and clinical research data available that we have now. Genes, of course, play a role in all cancer development, but as I have learned from Dr. Campbell, "Genes do not determine disease on their own. They function only by being activated or expressed. And nutrition plays a critical role in determining which genes, good and bad, are expressed."

As I mentioned earlier, this emerging knowledge has empowered me to make drastic changes in my own behavior and has motivated me to create a career helping other people understand the mounting scientific proof of the relationship between nutrition and the development of cancer and its progression.

With this well-researched connection between PC (most cancers for that matter) and diet, the medical oncological community has a long overdue, vital responsibility to assist their patients on becoming educated about using evidence-based nutrition as another strategic weapon on cancer.

Now is the time for the diet-disease connection to be acknowledged and addressed by the western medical community. Dr. Donald Abrams of UCSF in 2015 published an editorial in the Journal of Clinical Oncology stating the exact same opinion. "It's no longer acceptable to have your doctor give you the advice to 'eat better' and 'lose weight' in order to improve your health outcome." Dr. Abrams further states, "As oncologists become more aware of these undeniable associations, it becomes a critical part of our job to be able to answer patients' questions about nutrition during and after cancer treatment and not default to the unhelpful 'it doesn't really matter, eat what you want' which is not in the best interest of the patient."

I don't expect my oncologist to have a deep knowledge and education in evidence-based nutrition, but I DO expect more guidance than throw away quotes that mean nothing and have no effect in regard to what you put into your body on a daily basis. Today's oncologist should come to patient meetings with a minimum of a basic understanding of nutrition as it relates to cancer along with suggested internet links on nutrition and cancer as well as a specific recommendation of an integrative oncologist or nutritionist who has extensive experience in the field.

And this is beginning to happen, albeit not fast enough.

The Prostate Cancer Research Institute (PCRI) was founded by Dr. Mark Scholz, with the mission to improve the quality of prostate cancer patients' and caregivers' lives by empowering them to manage their prostate cancer through education. They hold an annual conference in Los Angeles and nutrition concerns are always on the agenda. Dr. Scholz recommends a "vegetarian diet" for PC patients (https://secure.pcri.org/np/clients/pcri/login.jsp?forwardedFromSecureDomain=1).

The Prostate Cancer Foundation (PCF), a non-profit you may be a member of, has recently released a lifestyle and dietary guideline for men diagnosed with prostate cancer (https://www.pcf.org/wp-content/uploads/2016/10/PCF_HW_Guide.pdf).

Created with the help of Harvard TH Chan School of Public Health and UCSF, the basic premise of the guideline is to eat a whole food, plant-based diet. My only concern with the PCF guideline is the recommendation of eating fish as well as to consume olive oil, both of which I will address later.

The MD Anderson Cancer Center, considered the world leader in the standard of cancer care, now recommends a whole-food, plant-based diet and includes it in their nutritional guidelines (https://www.mdanderson.org/documents/Departments-and-Divisions/Clinical-Nutrition/Nutrition-Basics-for-Patients-and-Caregivers.pdf) that are mailed and emailed to ALL of their patients.

The American Institute of Cancer Research has also recently released a "Heal Well Guide" with basically the same message: "At least two-thirds of your plate should be filled with whole-plant-based foods." When I read the "at least," I interpret this to mean "eat as many plant foods as possible, right up to 100% based on the best available evidence to date."

The updated guidelines with an emphasis on plant-based eating for cancer care are a big step in the right direction, but I believe we can do an even better job of utilizing nutritional intervention for PC by making BIG changes in our diets, and that is what I chose to do. It is also recommended by the experts. A PC diagnosis is a major wake-up call, and this is NOT the time to make timid and minor tweaks to our diets. In my opinion, the science supports going to 100% plant-based food as a nutritional adjunct to standard PC care.

Chapter 28 - Digging Deeper

So, why not consume a plant-based diet, lose weight, reduce your risk of PC, AND improve your odds of a long and healthy survival if you do have PC? I can't come up with any reason except the inability to engage in changing lifelong eating behaviors. Here is the bottom line: There is only ONE diet that has been proven effective over the long term for losing weight and keeping it off: A WFPB diet, minimizing or eliminating all processed and animal foods.

~ ~ ~

Expert Analysis / Behavior Change
Dr. Neil Barnard, PCRM

> We see lots of people here both in our clinic and in our research studies, and we find that there are certain things the human animal needs in order to make change. You have to understand why you're making the change, what's in it for you, and see a pathway forward. You have to make it kind of easy and maybe a little bit fun. People will change!

Expert Analysis / Behavior Change
Dr. Alan Goldhamer, TrueNorth Health Center

> The only real cure for cancer is prevention, but once you have a condition like prostate cancer, it is manageable. The

goal is to manage the condition, so you live a long and healthy life. The concept of a "cure" is misleading. We believe health results from healthful living.

The best motivators for behavioral change are pain, disability, and fear of death. Debilitating pain is fabulous. That will drive people to do extremely radical things like eat a plant-based diet, exercise, and go to bed on time. It's amazing what people will do if the pain is bad enough. The problem with pain is that when it goes away, people start deciding they are well again, and then they go back to the behavior that got them there in the first place, and it all comes raging back. Mark Twain said, "Denial is not just a river in Egypt," and I think what he was thinking about was people trying to make behavioral change. Trying to get people to change their behavior is very difficult. It is very hard for people to give up their addictions. If a person is an alcoholic and someone tells him or her, "Your life sucks because you are a drunk," they don't say, "Oh, it's the alcohol? I had no idea! Thank you so much! I just won't drink anymore." No way. They'll tell you to mind your own

Chapter 28 - Digging Deeper

business because they don't want to hear about it.

If you try to explain to people that what they are putting into their mouths is affecting their health, it's very difficult for them because all their lives they are told diet doesn't matter. If they go to a physician, the doctor usually will say, "Diet doesn't matter, eat whatever you want."

If you're a female and you lose a bunch of weight, and you go to your doctor, your doctor doesn't say, "Good for you! You've adopted a whole-food, plant-based diet, and have begun exercising." The doctor might think, *Well, you might have colon cancer, or you have developed an eating disorder, or you're a drug addict, or a combination of all of it because my experience is that nobody loses a bunch of weight and keeps it off unless they are dying of cancer or have developed an eating disorder or have a drug addiction.*

My experience and observation after more than nine years of research on how plant-based nutrition is a critical step in treating metabolic diseases such as PC are that people WILL change their behavior, but usually only after life-threatening conditions arise such as obesity and diabetes. We see the light bulb come on and we see people commit to change, just like I did. We get emails every day from people who have attended our courses letting us know their success in moving to a healthier diet. The preconceived notion by many medical experts that people will not change their behavior, especially as it relates to diet, is outdated, presumptive, and dangerous. Mindy and I have proven it WRONG ourselves.

Dr. Barnard also pointed out most cohort and randomized studies of plant-based nutrition to date have had marginal, and in some cases, disappointing results as far as chronic disease outcomes are concerned. Dr. Barnard, along with many other experts, believe this is due to the fact the differences in diet comparison groups in many of these massive cohort studies are relatively small. A perfect example of this can be found in the "Women's Health Initiative" and what they perceived as negative findings from some studies in breast cancer. Dr. Barnard stated:

> "The Women's Health Initiative" was this massive study, very expensive, and they brought in 10s of thousands of women and randomized them into various groups, and then they looked at what happened to them, and the intervention groups had only marginal reductions in cancer risk. However, the diet they were

asked to follow had very moderate, marginal changes to what they were eating before. As a result, the results were pretty miniscule.

The takeaway, according to Dr. Barnard:

Make little changes, you get a little benefit. If you make moderate changes, you're going to get a moderate benefit. If you make huge dramatic changes, you're likely to get dramatic results. That's why Dean Ornish did not say "Take the skin off your chicken," in his landmark study on PC and diet. He said, "Throw out the chicken, throw out the eggs, throw out the milk, beef, cheese, and fish."

And that is my message to you if you have been diagnosed with PC at ANY stage. NOW is the time to make big, dramatic changes to your lifestyle and diet if you expect to see and feel noticeable improvements in your health and outcome. Just GO ALL THE WAY! What's the risk or downside of this? From a health perspective, my experience has been there is only upside.

Summary

1. Don't expect your medical team to be experts in nutrition. Ask for and expect guidance from an evidence-based nutritionist or dietician. Don't accept throw-away answers to crucial questions.

2. A cancer diagnosis is an opportunity for positive behavioral change.
3. Make small changes—get small results. Big changes result in big results.

CHAPTER 29
WHO GETS PROSTATE CANCER AND WHY?

Health is not valued 'till sickness comes.

— Thomas Fuller

Following is a quick summary of my analysis and conclusion that prostate cancer is primarily a lifestyle-driven disease (at least in my case):

Let's start with who does and does not get PC. The longest-lived people on planet earth have been studied and documented by Dan Buettner, the author of the bestseller, *The Blue Zones.* Buettner and the *National Geographic Society* identified five locations around the planet where people (including us guys) routinely live into their 90s and 100s. Included in this elite group of healthy older populations are the Seventh Day Adventists in Loma Linda, CA, where they have a large community presence. Central and core to each of these well-studied populations, including the Adventists, is a foundational adherence to a whole-foods, plant-based diet. Every single one. There is no documented longest-lived society that eats a western diet, a Standard American Diet, a high-meat diet, a high-protein diet, or a high-fat diet. None. Zero.

Another great example of traditional minimally processed plant-based nutrition being central to long health are the people of Okinawa, Japan, who eat their traditional diet and who are also one of the Blue Zones identified by Mr. Buettner. Of course, they get cancer and other chronic diseases, but at much lower rates than we do in the US. According to Dan Buettner, they suffer one fifth the rate of heart disease, and a quarter the rate of breast and prostate cancer.[1]

A traditional Okinawan meal is miso soup, stir-fry veggies with seaweed, and green tea. Generally speaking, it is a low-calorie, low-fat, high-carbohydrate diet (just like all other documented longest-lived societies' diets). The average protein content of a meal in a traditional Okinawa meal is around 10%. Compare that to around 35% for the Standard American Diet. In addition to lower rates of all chronic diseases, the massive benefit of the Okinawa lifestyle and diet of fresh vegetables along with sweet potatoes with every meal turns out to be the highest life expectancies on the planet: 90 for women, and 84 for men. Compare that with the US: 81 for women and 76 for men. Additionally, there are over 400 centenarians in Okinawa.

The Okinawans do eat meat, of course, mostly in the form of fish, but traditionally, only for special occasions and certain holidays. Meat is NOT on the table for

Chapter 29 - Who Gets Prostate Cancer and Why?

breakfast, lunch, and dinner every single day like it was in my home.

Another point worth noting: Up until the early 20th century, the Okinawans calorie consumption came from one primary source: The Japanese sweet potato along with a diet of primarily millet, rice, and barley cultivation. Simple, simple, simple.

Dr. T. Colin Campbell's ground-breaking research, highlighted in his book, *The China Study,* showed the modern western world that cancer, heart disease, diabetes, and the rest are not uniformly present in all populations. This twenty-year study was conducted by the Chinese Academy of Preventive Medicine, Cornell University, and the University of Oxford. It examined mortality rates from cancer and other chronic diseases from 1973 to 1975. Considered the "Grand Prix" of nutritional research at the time, this comprehensive analysis of 65,000 people in 65 different counties in China revealed that diseases of the "Western World" tended to cluster together in certain areas where meat consumption was higher than the national average. In the entire country of China, the closer people came to an all plant-based diet, the lower their risk for chronic disease, including PC.

Dr. Campbell thought his research would change the course of human nutrition. How could it not? Wouldn't everyone want to move towards a plant-based diet and reap the results? Well, I don't think the world was ready for *The China Study* when it was published in 2004, and Dr. Campbell endured (and continues to do so) vicious attacks from the animal food industries and their paid professionals.

~ ~ ~

Expert Analysis / Cancer Prevention and Treatment
Dr. T. Colin Campbell

> There are 28 institutes at NIH, and not one is dedicated to nutrition. Doctors don't get the research money that they deserve to learn more about nutrition, so the system is stuck in place. Nutrition didn't get the attention that it deserved. There are 130 medical categories that we work with. Not one is called nutrition. Not one out of 130. So, the doctors aren't trained and they can't be reimbursed. They have to do it on their own time. What we have now is the dark ages in the context of medicine. It's not what it could be, what it should be. And you can see it kind of peeling off the layers of knowledge and the developments going through the ages how this happened, that happened, this happened. And it got to a place where the medical system is almost like a religion.
>
> In my mind, it is not just about prevention. The bigger story is about treatment. We always divided prevention and treatment. That's part of medical history. But it turns out prevention is treatment. But

treatment is where the money is and the leftovers, you know, just got involved in prevention. Prevention and treatment are one and the same. A WFPBD can, to some extent, prevent future disease. When it's done right, it becomes easy treatment, and it does more than all the pills and procedures combined. That's the future.

I'm very passionate about the idea of science. I think there's a synonym for the word science. It's called integrity. And if one is to follow the science, they're following facts—and trying to discover facts, you always have to be prepared to be wrong. That is just as important as trying to be right. It's the idea of preparing to be wrong and accepting it or inviting it. You have to invite comment, and then have a discussion in a civil manner, of course. I like science in the classical sense. Modern-day science, especially in academia, has been corrupted. We're limited as scientists because a lot of academic freedom is at a 10-year decline and almost gone. Additionally, the funding that has traditionally come from independent government bodies is now becoming a corporate sector.

~ ~ ~

Expert Analysis / Cancer Prevention and Treatment
Dr. Michael Greger, Nutritionfacts.org:
Cancer Prevention and Treatment

Cancer prevention and cancer treatment are the same things. In the first few decades, when you have cancer, you don't even know about it. These epithelial glandular tumors like colon cancer, breast cancer, prostate cancer, and lung cancer take decades to develop. So, between that first DNA mutation and when you're actually diagnosed, that's decades long, so every single day, you have cancer you don't know about. People get diagnosed with cancer, and they think if they didn't have cancer yesterday, how do they have cancer today? No, you've had cancer for decades.

Every single day where you thought you were preventing cancer by eating a healthy diet, you're actually treating it with the hope that it will never go far enough, and you won't get diagnosed with it in your lifetime. Every single day, tiny little microscopic tumors are rising, getting decimated by our immune system. That's why we cannot wait until diagnosis, and even after diagnosis, it's the same process. You are preventing further progression.

~ ~ ~

Chapter 29 - Who Gets Prostate Cancer and Why?

This is the situation at hand. Now, most funding for nutritional research is conducted by corporations that want to prove some sort of efficacy of a new drug or by the junk and animal food industries that want their products to have a "health halo."

The China Study research revealed that up until very recent economic development in China, most of its massive rural population have traditionally eaten a plant-centered diet which is coupled with 120 times LESS prostate cancer than men in the US.[2,3]

You may be thinking that the people of the "Blue Zones" and the rural Chinese have unique genes that provide them with better longevity. NOT SO: There are also two subsequent research data sets to consider:

> When these same populations begin to adopt the modern western diet of processed foods, eggs, dairy, and meat, their rates of cancer, including prostate cancer, as well as all of the other chronic diseases associated with this type of diet, begin to go up.
>
> Additionally, several population migration studies have clearly demonstrated that when people migrate from an area that has a low incidence of chronic disease and PC to the US, their disease rates, including PC, catch up to ours within one generation.[4]

> This is currently happening in almost all of the Blue Zones and is particularly of note for the Okinawans. Dr. Michael Greger, in his landmark book, *How Not to Die,* explains that since World War II, Japanese consumption of eggs has gone up by 7x, dairy by 20x, and 9x for meat. Coinciding with this rapid acceleration of animal food consumption, PC rates in Japan have shot up by 25X.[5]

~ ~ ~

Mindy and I recently visited another Blue Zone, Nicoya, Costa Rica. We wanted to see for ourselves how these folks lived and what they ate. As we drove into the main part of downtown Nicoya, we noticed a brand new Kentucky Fried Chicken (directly across the street from the new McDonald's that had just opened up on Main Street). The line was out the door. Everybody loves fried chicken. I grew up on it.

As I do my own mental recall of food consumption, my childhood, early adulthood, and most of my adult years of dairy consumption was, well, tremendous. Whole milk and sometimes whipped cream was a standard on Captain Crunch cereal through high school. Every night in our home was ice cream night. I also loved to make milk shakes at least four or five times a week. Then, in college, my roommates and I would consume a GALLON of Breyer's ice cream in the evenings after eating dinner at the local barbeque joint. My adult years up to age 52 were pretty much the same. Cheese was an obsession of mine for most of my life and was one of the last of the dairy products I finally gave up. If you feel addicted to cheese, there is a reason. The casomorphin in cheese has an addictive quality, just like...morphine! Dr. Neal Barnard has written an excellent book entitled *The Cheese Trap* that outlines just how addictive and dangerous cheese actually is. Dr. Barnard summarizes that it is high in calories, contains concentrated amounts of casein, is high in saturated fat and cholesterol, and is packed with excessive sodium. I love cheese. However, it's no longer on my plate and has been replaced with nutritional yeast, an excellent and healthy substitute with a cheesy flavor. For special occasions, I always try to have or bring a really well-made nut-based cheese to social events. It's amazing how far plant-based cheeses have come, and it's fun trying new ones. Just a few cautions:

1. Plant-based cheeses are high in fat, so use sparingly.
2. Read the label! Most commercial vegan cheeses have a ton of added liquid processed fat in the form of soybean, rice, and canola oils. All of these polyunsaturated free fats are very high in Omega-6 fatty acids that are considered to be proinflammatory. Make sure you buy an artisanal vegan cheese that has no added free fats, just the whole nuts which are usually cashews.

Enough on cheese for now...

Summary

1. Genes play a minor role in cancer initiation and development. Don't feed your cancer!
2. From a nutritional perspective, cancer prevention is treatment.
3. The modern western diet is the primary driver of all chronic disease

CHAPTER 30
CANCER AND OBESITY

Obesity is a normal response to an abnormal environment.

— Dr. Michael Greger

According to the AICR, one of the strongest findings from their continuous research updates is the link between excess body fat and cancer. According to the AICR, research worldwide calculated that approximately 117,000 cancer cases in the United States each year are linked to excess body fat.[1]

Specific to PC, researchers examined the association between obesity and risk of low and high-grade cancers using biopsies from the "REDUCE" study ("REDUCE"— A Clinical Research Study to Reduce the Incidence of Prostate Cancer in Men Who Are at Increased Risk"). In the study, it was found that obesity is directly linked to an increased risk of PC recurrence, aggressive PC, and death from PC.[2] Additionally, a 2004 study published in the *Journal of Clinical Oncology* discovered statistically significantly higher rates of aggressive PC in obese men in addition to higher recurrence after surgery.[3]

The issue with fat is that it is not inert as had been previously thought. Recent research has shown that fat in our bodies is busy producing hormones such as leptin in addition to secreting inflammation-promoting cytokines, a type of signaling protein usually in white blood cells. Cancer cells can respond to host-derived cytokines that promote growth, attenuate apoptosis, and facilitate invasion and metastasis. Furthermore, excess body fat, especially visceral body fat around the abdomen, has been shown to increase estrogen production, impair immunity, and increase insulin resistance which raises insulin and other growth factors that can promote cancer.[4]

On a very personal note, a very obese friend and business associate of mine, the same age as me, was diagnosed with metastatic PC in 2011, the same year as me. He had a huge heart and a wonderful soul, but he could not control his addiction to fried animal and processed food even after his diagnosis. He died one year later.

What's the best way to avoid or eliminate obesity for a lifetime? A low-fat, whole-foods, plant-based diet! Dr. Greger outlines the details of the "Adventist Health Study 2" in his book, *How Not to Diet:*

> The largest study ever to compare the obesity rates of those eating plant-based diets was published in North America. Meat eaters topped the charts with an average body mass index (BMI) of 28.8—close to being obese. Flexitarians (people

who ate meat more on a weekly basis rather than daily) did better at a BMI of 27.3, but were still overweight. With a BMI of 26.3, pesco-vegetarians (people who avoid all meat except fish) did better still. Even U.S. vegetarians tend to be marginally overweight, coming in at 25.7. The only dietary group found to be of ideal weight were those eating strictly plant-based (the "vegans"), whose BMI averaged 23.6.[5]

After that, the BROAD study, a randomized control trial, investigated the use of a WFPBD in a community for obesity diabetes and heart disease in New Zealand. The study completed a randomized controlled clinical trial of 65 participants presenting with early signs of metabolic syndrome (high-risk factors for chronic disease, including obesity). It showed after six months that a WFPB diet was optimum for weight loss. According to the researchers, "this research achieved greater weight loss at six and twelve months than any other trial that does not limit energy intake or mandate regular exercise."[6]

It worked for me, taking my weight (not to mention my cholesterol, triglycerides, and blood pressure) down quickly and FOREVER. When I dove into implementing plant-based nutrition after the *"China Study* Plane Flight," my weight went from 176 down to my current weight of 135 pounds in less than six months. It has never changed on my plant-based diet (except during prolonged fasting). My energy level is through the roof even after being diagnosed with advanced PC nine years ago. Did I mention how delicious my diet is?

Summary

1. Obesity puts us at increased risk of developing PC, as well as recurrent and aggressive PC.
2. WFPB eaters, on an average, have lower BMIs compared to SAD eaters.
3. Lose the weight via WFPB nutrition to improve your odds of a good outcome. Nothing tastes better than vibrant health.

CHAPTER 31
CLINICAL TRIALS

Every time you eat or drink, you are either feeding disease or fighting it.

— Heather Morgan

There are now scores of randomized controlled clinical trials, considered the "gold standard" of research, demonstrating that transitioning to a WFPB diet can actually reverse heart disease[1] and diabetes.[2]

Dr. Dean Ornish and Dr. Caldwell Esselstyn have both completed long-term elegantly designed randomized controlled trials that have proven beyond any doubt that heart disease progression can not only be halted in its tracks but can also be reversed, effectively curing late-stage heart disease.[3] Both Dr. Esselstyn's and Dr. Ornish's programs are now covered by most major insurance companies.

Dr. Esselstyn's study results were published at five, twelve, and sixteen years, and updated even beyond twenty years. According to Dr. E:

"The compliant patients' angina diminished and largely disappeared; they achieved and maintained cholesterol goals, and angiographic evidence showed their disease had selectively reversed. Most importantly, they survived. My recent book, *Prevent and Reverse Heart Disease*, updates the study beyond 21 years, making it the longest of its type. Those patients told by expert cardiologists 20 years ago that they had less than a year to live who are alive and well in 2007 are a particularly compelling story."[4]

Regarding diabetes, Dr. Neal Barnard, Founder and Director of the Physicians Committee for Responsible Medicine, has completed pioneering research demonstrating both the cause of diabetes (fat deposits in our cells) as well as the ability to clear this "intramyocellular fat" from our cells improving insulin resistance and reversing diabetes via (you guessed it) a low-fat WFPB diet.[5]

And most pertinent to you and me, a handful of quality randomized controlled trials have demonstrated a WFPB diet's ability to REVERSE PSA acceleration and PC growth in early-stage prostate cancer. Dr. Dean Ornish has shown that an intensive diet change can indeed stop and REVERSE the growth of early-stage prostate cancer in his randomized controlled trial.[6]

In 2005, he recruited 93 men with early state PC and randomly divided them into two groups. The experimental group patients were prescribed an intensive lifestyle program that included a vegan diet supplemented with soy (1 daily serving of tofu plus 58 gm of a fortified soy protein powdered beverage), fish oil (3 gm daily), vitamin E (400 IU daily), selenium (200 mcg daily) and vitamin C (2 gm daily), moderate aerobic exercise (walking 30 minutes 6 days weekly), stress management techniques (gentle yoga-based stretching, breathing, meditation, imagery and progressive relaxation for a total of 60 minutes daily) and participation in an hour-long support group once a week to enhance adherence to the intervention. The diet was fruits, vegetables, whole grains, legumes, and soy products, low in simple carbohydrates, and with approximately 10% of calories from fat. This is the definition of a truly low-fat diet. The Centers for Disease Control (CDC) as of 2018 estimates the SAD diet is approximately 30% fat[7], so this is a significant reduction in fat consumption and is important to note.

I think the key component of this study was that, not only was the experimental group Instructed to eat the diet coupled with intensive personal counseling, the food was actually delivered to their door each day assuring adherence. The control group was given no instruction to change diet. After one year, PSA levels had decreased in the group that had implemented the diet change. In the control group, PSA levels continued to rise, and some of the participants actually had to abandon the trial for surgery or radiation treatment. Specifically, serum PSA decreased an average of 0.25

ng/ml or 4% of the baseline average in the experimental group. It showed an average increase of 0.38 ng/ml or 6% of the baseline average in the control group.

Additionally, changes in prostate cancer cell growth (LNCaP) from baseline to 12 months were significantly different between the groups, showing more favorable changes in the experimental group. Serum from the experimental group patients inhibited LNCaP cell growth by 70%, whereas serum from control group patients inhibited growth by only 9%. C-reactive protein (CRP), the most common measurement of inflammation, decreased more in the experimental group. There were no significant differences between the groups in serum testosterone or in apoptosis (programmed cell death).[8]

Dr. Dean Ornish's work is the gold standard of scientific research: a randomized controlled trial. Granted, this was a small study, and with early-stage PC, but the statistical significance of reversing PSA velocity in existing cancer with a plant-based diet is powerful. It turns out there is even more research demonstrating the power of WFPB diets on existing or recurrent PC. I used Dr. Michael Greger's website, nutritionfacts.org. as one of the primary tools to find these studies. It's an incredible website with access to deep research.

There are only a few completed quality RCTs on nutritional intervention and PC progression, but each has demonstrated that "leaning to the green" (moving more TOWARDS a WFPBD) has the ability to slow or even

Chapter 31 – Clinical Trials

reverse advanced, metastatic PC. And we say this in our One Day to Wellness Program… "Leaning to the green is the way to go."

In 2012 A group of Harvard researchers performed a study to see if just adding more fruits and vegetables to study subjects' diets and moving them away from processed and animal foods would have an impact on prostate cancer growth. Thirty-six men with definitive PC and their partners were randomly assigned to either a series of plant-based cooking and mindfulness classes or a control group with no instructions. The experimental group showed a significant reduction in saturated fat intake as well as a reduction in animal protein along with an increase in plant-based protein. The mean PSA doubling time for the intervention group was substantially longer at the three-month follow-up visit than that of the control group.[9] It looks like just the simple effort to "lean to the green" can have a significant impact on PC progression.

In 2006, Dr. Gordon Saxe and his team of researchers at the Moore's Cancer Center and School of Medicine at the University of California San Diego completed the "UCSD Healthy Men Study." This was a pre-post pilot clinical trial in which each patient served as his own control. Its purpose was to determine whether a plant-based dietary intervention, reinforced by stress reduction, could effect a major dietary change and influence the progression of recurrent PC. This small study demonstrated that dietary intervention may actually slow or halt

PC growth AFTER RECURRENCE.[10] This small and relatively short study (ten patients, six months) focused on PSA levels in response to a plant-based diet and mindfulness training. Results? The plant-based diet and stress reduction intervention significantly reduced PSA acceleration and even reversed it in four of the ten patients. Nine of the ten saw their PSA slow down. The median time it took for men's PSA levels to double increased from 11.9 months at pre-study to 112.3 months at intervention. WHAT? This is huge! According to Dr. Saxe, "The magnitude of the effect of these findings is the strongest observed to date among dietary and nutritional interventions in this patient population."

Again, the key component to the outcome of this study was the experimental group's adherence to the low-fat vegan diet. In order to guarantee compliance, Dr. Saxe and his team made sure the patients actually ate the food.

~ ~ ~

Expert Analysis—Dr. Gordon Saxe

> We put these men in a full-court press. First of all, I got very friendly with a couple of the urologists here at UCSD and the urologists hand-picked eligible subjects, and then they reinforced the message. Plus, these guys, their wives were like, with a rolling pin over there, "Honey, you're going to do this." And

Chapter 31 – Clinical Trials

their cardiologists were telling them the same thing. You got hypercholesterolemia; you got heart disease, whatever. You need to do the same damn set of challenges. And we made it the path of least resistance for these men to follow the diet. We conducted cooking classes, but the wives came more than the husbands did. The wives became our fifth caller. They became the ones who saved the husbands from themselves, put the food on the table in front of them, and basically got them to change.

Additionally, they had counselling at the beginning, midpoint, and end. I think it was three counselling sessions per person. And they had some telephone follow-ups with the dietitian as well. So, they had the message reinforced that way. They came to weekly cooking classes in the first month, and we rented the International Centre on campus. I hired some macrobiotic chefs, and they made these incredibly wonderful plant-based meals. While they were finishing, they would demo some of the cooking things. And then, while they were finishing up the cooking, I would take them into this beautiful living room, and I and another friend of mine from Pacific College, the Chinese medicine school, taught them yoga, tai chi, and meditation. And then they'd come together; the meal would be ready. Then we'd sit family style at a bunch of tables. They had a community dinner together.

They really did form a community. At the very end of that study, we celebrated the six-month mark. One of the people in this study was very wealthy, and he opened up his home, and we had a wonderful meal there, we had a big party, and gave gifts to each other. And, you know, it's a real celebration. By then, I had the final, crude data to share with them because I had just finished all the last set of measurements, and the study was successful.

Again, WOW. Statistically significant and actionable outcomes. You don't need any more studies! Just DO IT. And as the above studies indicate, to get significant outcomes, you HAVE to make BIG changes. My advice: Don't nibble around the edges of changing your diet. GO ALL THE WAY. Do you really want to go from 5 eggs a week to 2? Have you ever known anyone who was successful in quitting smoking by committing to smoking only half a pack a day instead of a whole pack? This is torture that you don't have to endure. Commit, and you won't be sorry.

Chapter 31 – Clinical Trials

Finally, I want to discuss the most recent randomized clinical trial investigating: "The effect of a behavioral intervention to increase vegetable consumption on cancer regression among men with early-stage PC," also known as The MEAL Randomized Clinical trial.[11] The study was posted on JAMA and the Prostate Cancer Foundation's Website in March of 2020 and was funded by the National Cancer Institute (NCI). The important point to remember for this study is it was targeting the "effect of a behavioral change intervention." It was NOT an interventional trial changing what their subject's ate. It was simply a study of the suggestion to eat more fruits and vegetables.

It was a randomized clinical trial conducted at 91 US urology and medical oncology clinics that enrolled 478 men aged 50 to 80 years with biopsy-proven prostate adenocarcinoma grade group = 1 in those <70 years and ≤2 in those ≥70 years, stage cT2a or less, and PSA level less than 10 ng/mL. It was a 24-month study from January 2013 to August 2017.

The intervention group patients were randomized to a counseling behavioral intervention by telephone promoting consumption of seven or more daily vegetable servings (MEAL intervention; n=237). That's it? One group got some phone calls over a two-year period counseling patients to increase vegetable consumption. That's it.

The control group received the Prostate Cancer Foundation eating guide which is a detailed brochure about diet and prostate cancer (n = 241) which is essentially guidance to EAT A PLANT-BASED DIET. Fundamentally, the same message was given to both groups with the only difference being one got phone calls and the other got a glossy pamphlet!

The conclusion of the MEAL study was "men with early-stage prostate cancer managed with active surveillance. A behavioral intervention that increased vegetable consumption did not significantly reduce the risk of prostate cancer progression. The findings do not support use of this intervention to decrease prostate cancer progression in this population, although the study may have been underpowered to identify a clinically important difference. PSA progression was essentially the same for both the intervention and control groups."

Even the authors acknowledge that the study was "underpowered."

Think about this. Do you know ANY men between the ages of 50 and 80 years old who have been eating the SAD diet for most of their lives and have even attempted to transition to eating a plant-based diet based on a phone discussion or reading a pamphlet for that matter? I don't. This is one of the most difficult behaviors to implement, even incrementally change. My experience has been that older men (like myself) are the least likely subset of our population to make changes to their diet. That's been my direct anecdotal experience helping people move in this direction for the last 10 years.

Chapter 31 – Clinical Trials

Phone calls without direct human interaction are likely to be non-motivational, compared to a face-to-face visit with a doctor who believes in dietary interventions along with follow-up and motivational visits. I also am not surprised by the unimpressive results. Furthermore, it looks like there was no instruction as to how to shop for and prepare the vegetables.

Also, there was no documentation of what these subjects WERE ACTUALLY EATING. WHAT? How do we know if telling them to eat fruits and veggies had an impact without knowing if they even ate them?

And most importantly, we can only presume all the men in both groups continued eating their usual meat and dairy products throughout the study, filled with growth-promoting sex hormones which we know stimulates the men's IGF-1 production and accelerates cancer growth.

We know it's not enough to just ADD more veggies to a crappy, disease-promoting diet. We need to eliminate the known disease-promoting foods as well! Effective dietary therapy requires BOTH the cessation of eating animal products AND the eating of more vegetables according to every expert on the subject.

With public funding for nutritional research already as tight as it is, I simply do not understand why the NCI would fund such a limp comparison of SUGGESTIONS and think they would have any significant outcome. This is a classic example of a poorly designed study that didn't produce meaningful results but which generated the usual I-told-you-so headlines. UGH.

So, we really have only three significant RCTs that have been performed on men with existing PC. Both the Ornish and Saxe studies were small, but each intervention was a commitment by the experimental group to eating an exclusively 100% plant-based diet with approximately 10% fat and NO ANIMAL PRODUCTS. Additionally, the meals were made for them and there were multiple group and one-on-one face-to-face consultations for both. Both of these studies showed statistically significant improvements, and sometimes reversal, in PSA velocity and cancer progression, in both recently diagnosed AND post-treatment recurrence.

Then we have this final third study, which is the largest of the three, but with no actual food intervention with the experimental group. As a result, there was probably little actual behavior change and, therefore, small or no change in PSA acceleration between the experimental and control group.

This study's results reinforce what Dr. Barnard emphasized throughout our discussion: "Make small changes, get small results. Make big changes, get big results!"

Summary

1. Be skeptical when investigating research. Look for large, government-funded population studies. Small studies funded by specific industries

Chapter 31 – Clinical Trials

investigating specific nutrients in specific foods are NOT a good source of scientific information.

2. PC RCTs are limited but clearly demonstrate that following a WFPB diet can slow the growth of early and recurrent stage PC.
3. This is not the time for "dipping your toes" into behavior change. Commit, dive in, and experience for yourself the power of plant-based nutrition.

CHAPTER 32
EATING PATTERNS AROUND THE GLOBE

Unbelievable as it may seem, one-third of all vegetables consumed in the United States come from just three sources: French fries, potato chips, and iceberg lettuce.

— Marion Nestle

Currently in China, the same story of a rapid upward trend of chronic disease and PC is unfolding just in the last decade. Increasing wealth and prosperity always comes with increased dietary consumption of processed foods, meat, dairy, and eggs. These large population diet changes always portend an increase in rates of cancer, heart disease, and diabetes within less than a decade.[1,2,3]

People who eat a plant-based diet generally live longer and suffer fewer chronic diseases, including PC.[4] Additionally, large epidemiological population studies, like the "Global Burden of Health Study," show that PC rates, along with ALL western chronic diseases are

MUCH higher in areas of the world that have long-established "western" style eating habits where meat, dairy, eggs, and ultra-processed foods take center stage on the plate.[5] These populations, as expected, cluster around the modern industrialized western world with the US at the top. We are #1! Conversely, the lowest reported levels of PC tend to occur in Asian countries, where traditional diets consist mostly of low-fat, plant-centered foods.

Here is a glaring example: The US has 10 times the rate of prostate cancer than that of Japan, but, when Japanese men move to the US and transition from their traditional soy-rich, low-fat, plant-based diet to the SAD diet, their prostate cancer rates catch up to ours within one generation.[6] Rates of other chronic diseases such as heart disease, diabetes, stroke, and Alzheimer's also cluster around countries that consume the western diet resulting in shorter lives.[7,8]

This clustering of chronic diseases has many implications for us men with PC as we are usually within the clusters! Heart disease continues to be the most common non-cancer cause of death for men with prostate cancer according to a recent publication in the medical journal, *Circulation.*[9]

And, because these chronic diseases cluster in people who eat the SAD diet, men diagnosed with PC also tend to have much higher rates of other common chronic conditions such as diabetes and stroke compared to the general US population.[10]

Additionally, a 2017 study published in the *British Journal of Cancer* followed a cohort of 7,637 men with early-stage, localized prostate cancer between 1998 and 2008, and found an 81% increased risk of heart failure (in men without preexisting conditions) when androgen deprivation therapy (ADT) was introduced.[11] This new research along with other collaborating studies makes an even STRONGER case for adopting a WFPB diet if you are on ADT because we know that a diet high in animal products, and red meat in particular, drastically increases the risk of heart disease.[12]

There is now a huge number of large cross-sectional studies (analyzing a large population in a snapshot of time, like Dr. Campbell's *China Study*) as well as cohort population studies following millions of people for decades which clearly demonstrate that the more a western diet is consumed, the higher the risk of being diagnosed and dying of these same clustered metabolic diseases, including PC. In 2007, the World Health Organization (WHO) along with the American Institute for Cancer Research (AICR) and the World Cancer Research Fund (WCRF) completed a meta-analysis of ALL the relevant research to date on diet and cancer and came to the following conclusions[13]:

> There is a clear correlation between meat consumption and many forms of cancer.
>
> Diets should be mostly of plant origin.
>
> Plant-based diets offer protection against heart disease and cancer.

These are considered to be the most experienced, unbiased, and well-informed nutritional scientists in the world. The next time someone questions or doubts you about eating a plant-based diet (I am making the assumption you already do, or are going to after reading this book!), ask them if they think they have a better handle on global nutrition than the expert scientists of the World Health Organization or the National Institute of Health.

In 2012, the T. H. Chan School of Public Health published the two largest nutritional studies ever conducted: "The Nurse's Health Study" which followed 120,000 women for 38 years and the "Health Professionals Follow-up Study" which followed 50,000 men for 32 years. Each of these massive studies concluded that "consuming processed and unprocessed red meat is associated with an increased risk of dying from cancer and heart disease and shortened life spans overall."[14]

"This study provides clear evidence that regular consumption of red meat, especially processed meat, contributes substantially to premature death," according to Dr. Frank Hu, one of the senior scientists involved in the study and a professor of nutrition at the Harvard School of Public Health.

People in the study who had the highest intake of red meat tended to die younger, and more often from cardiovascular disease and cancer. They also tended to weigh more, exercise less, smoke tobacco more, and drink more alcohol than healthier people in the study.

Yet even when the researchers compensated for the effects of an unhealthy lifestyle and mortality, meat remained associated with an earlier death in general.[15]

Currently, the largest ongoing nutritional cohort study ever conducted, the "NIH-AARP Diet and Health Study" which followed 500,000 people for decades, recently published their initial results: "Meat consumption is associated with an increased risk dying from cancer, heart disease, and premature death in general."[16] OK, that's brief and succinct. After the results were published by the National Institutes of Health (NIH), the American Medical Association (AMA) called for "a major reduction in total meat intake."[17]

Summary:

1. Animal flesh is not required in the human diet and has been directly linked to multiple cancers as well as heart disease.
2. There are no nutrients in animal-based foods that are not better provided by plants.
3. When you open up your refrigerator, you want to see a garden, not a morgue.

CHAPTER 33
IT'S THE FOOD

It's always been the food.

—Dr. Michael Klaper

The summary of evidence I have outlined is exactly what motivated ("compelled" might be a better word) me to make drastic changes to my lifestyle. The body of research is overwhelming. My own personal experience, as well as years of research and lecturing on the topic of making this transition, has proved to me that eating a low-fat WFPB diet is the optimal diet for human health and the optimal diet to treat PC. But to put the nail in the coffin, so to speak, let's drill down into the research on some specific foods that have been well studied for both their contribution to the development of PC as well as the progression of PC.

Dr. John McDougall has summarized extensive research on cancer and diet, and I have leveraged much of his work and observations in compiling this book and this chapter. I highly recommend going to his website as well as reading his recently published book, *The Starch Solution,* which outlines how the human population has survived and thrived throughout history, primarily eating a starch-based vegan diet. Dr. McDougall doesn't mince words and doesn't hesitate to confront the dairy, egg, beef, junk-food industries for their obvious attempts to obfuscate the mountain of research piling up on the dangers of the foods they produce. All of his blogs and videos are deeply researched and presented in easy-to-understand language for us civilians.

Milk and IGF-1

The EPIC (European Prospective Investigation into Cancer and Nutrition) study is one of the largest global cohort studies in the world, with 521,000 participants recruited from 10 European countries and followed for almost 15 years. This massive study analyzed a wide range of potential-risk factors, including lifestyle, diet, and genetics. The single most important risk factor identified for prostate cancer is an increased blood level of IGF-1[1,] a natural human growth hormone produced by the liver. After reaching adulthood, levels of IGF-1 should drop significantly until they reach almost zero. However, a lifelong diet high in processed foods, dairy, and animal products has been shown to increase IGF-1 and keep them above optimal adult levels. What does IGF-1 do? It sends the signal to GROW. What increases serum IGF-1? Animal foods, and animal protein, in particular, are the biggest culprits.[2]

Want to get rid of excessive IGF-1 that can continue to fuel the growth of prostate cancer? Simply stop consuming animal protein. As Dr. Greger points out in *How Not To Die,* only men who limit their intake of ALL animal protein, including fish, dairy, eggs, and meat, are able to get a significant drop in blood levels of IGF-1.[3]

Finally, another large ecologic (multi-country) study looked at mortality data from 1986 and found a strong correlation between milk consumption and prostate cancer deaths.[4]

EXPERT OPINION / IGF-1 and Cancer

Dr. Neal Barnard:

> I think we can make our bet, but what we obviously want to do is to take all of these food components out of the equation. In dairy products and cancer risk, my money is on IGF-1. When a person drinks milk, they get a very predictable rise in IGF-1 levels. And we know that IGF-1 is a very potent stimulus for not only prostate cancer cell growth but other forms of cancer as well.
>
> There are other mechanisms, such as vitamin D being involved. If you drink more milk, it oddly enough suppresses vitamin D activation, because there's so much calcium in the milk that the body reacts by saying, "What's all this calcium coming

in? I don't want to absorb quite so much." So, it reduces vitamin D activation. Vitamin D is a cancer preventer, and if you're a milk drinker, you are reducing your Vitamin D activation. At least, that's what we think. The Harvard researchers who did the "Physicians' Health Study" first, and then the "Health Professional Follow-Up Study" are saying, "I think it's the Vitamin D." But it could also be the IGF-1. Or it could be the fact that milk has a lot of calories, and cheese has even more, and that if you're eating these foods, you're going to gain weight, and weight gain is also associated with increased risk of cancer.

Plus, all the good stuff that's in fruits and vegetables is not in the milk. Milk is not a plant, and it doesn't have fiber. It doesn't have the huge cornucopia of antioxidants that are in vegetables and fruits. A tomato can brag about lycopene. Milk can say, "Well, at least we got calcium," but that does not help your prostate at all.

It's a little bit like tobacco, where it was clear by the 1950s that tobacco caused lung cancer. But to this day, it's not

Chapter 33 – It's the Food

entirely clear what it is in the tobacco smoke that really gets the blame for it. Is it the benzyl-8-purine, or is it something else? And what's pretty likely with tobacco is that it's several different things.

What is it in milk? Is it the fact it raises your IGF-1; is it the fact that it suppresses your anti-cancer defenses; is it the fact that it just doesn't have what your body needs? It may be all these things. The good news is, it doesn't matter. Just avoid it! Let the scientists sort that out. You just have to avoid it.

Most of us grew up with this notion that animal products are really nutritious. That Fargo, North Dakota, view of the world where I grew up was people are starving in China, and here we've got protein! The truth, though is, the animal products are very skewed in that although they have a lot of protein, they have a lot of fat and a lot of cholesterol. They don't have that balance of all the nutrients that make up the plant kingdom. Vitamin C, well, it doesn't have any. Fiber, it doesn't have any of that at all. All animal foods are really generally poor in these nutritional components.

So, the point I'm making is that we grew up with these meat-centered diets, thinking that they're very nutritious, but it turns out they're really nutrient-poor. So you grow up with whatever vulnerability you may inherit. Your cancer defenses may be strong, may not be strong. Your likelihood of having a genetic mutation may be big or small.

It's very likely that the real drivers of prostate cancer in particular and several other cancers have nothing to do with genetics, and instead, it's all about the environment that allows those genes to express themselves.

And we've seen this with other conditions too. We see it with Alzheimer's disease. There are genes for Alzheimer's, clear-cut genes for Alzheimer's. But even if you have those genes, if you eat in a certain way, you can reduce your risk. There are genes for diabetes that runs up and down family trees. If you eat a certain way, it's likely you will get type two diabetes.

None of this is perfect. You can follow a great diet and still get cancer. But you don't want to play those odds. You want to unload the gun, not play that play. Well, you can smoke a pack a day and never get lung cancer. The majority of smokers do not get lung cancer. But so many do—it's just too risky.

EXPERT OPINION / IGF-1 and Cancer

Dr. Michael Greger:

> There's enough research in my view that, if you have prostate cancer, you'd have to be crazy not to get with the WFPB program. Even before all the data was available, Japan began to Westernize their diet. When dairy consumption shot up, there goes prostate cancer just skyrocketing through the roof. And we're talking fatal prostate cancer, dying with our tumors and from our tumors. The data is clear that with animal product consumption, probably through an IGF-1 mechanism, we are increasing the rate of growth, proliferation, invasiveness of cancer—all promoted by IGF-1, which is a consequence of animal protein consumption.

Eggs and dairy have been identified as two of the most likely food suspects we have with the diet and prostate cancer connection. The "Health Professionals

Follow Up Study," which followed 48,000 men, found that those who ate 2.5 or more eggs per week had an 81% increase in risk of getting lethal prostate cancer compared to those who ate less than half an egg per week.[5]

For my entire life, all 62 years of it, cow's milk has been marketed to our population and our children as an essential food that gives us sufficient calcium to build strong bones. And with the USDA's unwavering financial support, the dairy industry has become one of the largest food-producing industries in the US and the Western World.[6]

As early as 1999, cow's milk consumption has been consistently associated with a higher risk of developing PC.[7] Additionally, the Harvard School of Public Health cited in a recent review that high consumption of dairy was linked to a 50% increase in the risk of developing PC.[8] The association has just grown stronger in recent years.

Dr. Barnard also notes that dairy products have been implicated in increasing your risk of death from PC. In a study published in the *International Journal of Cancer*, researchers monitored the dairy intake of 926 men diagnosed with PC as part of the "Physician's Health Study" for 10 years. Those consuming three or more servings of dairy products a day increased their risk for overall death by 76% and had a 141% higher risk of death due to PC compared to those who consumed less than one serving.[9]

IGF-1 increases dramatically with an increase in animal protein consumption in general as previously outlined, but milk takes the gold medal.[10] Cow's milk has the ability to increase IGF-1 in our body by up to 10% just by consuming what the dairy industry recommends.

High levels of IGF-1 as an adult are associated with an increased risk of most cancers commonly diagnosed in the US, including PC.[11] On the flip side, it turns out men who consume a mostly plant-based vegan diet have about 10% lower IGF-1 levels compared to men who eat the SAD diet.[12]

Dr. Greger, in *How Not To Die* also points out that a host of case-control and cohort studies have determined that consumption of cow's milk is definitely a risk factor for PC.[13,14] In addition to increasing IGF-1 levels, dairy products may also drive PC growth because of the high levels of other hormones in milk, such as estrogen, and by the extremely high levels of saturated fat, which increase insulin levels, fat storage, and inflammation.

More on Meat

I grew up eating steak and hamburgers. Every Sunday night was "Sunday Night Supper" at my grandparent's house where a giant slab of a cow was grilled and served to everyone in my family. Other nights of the week, it was pork chops, or hamburger, or fried chicken. Meat was always center stage on our plates for breakfast, lunch, and dinner, just like everyone else I knew. I wish we knew then what we know now:

> High consumption of red meat (and dairy) is linked to a 2x elevation in risk of metastatic PC.

The data was gathered from the "Harvard Health Professional's Follow-Up Study," and included 51,529 men and concluded that "Intake of red meat and dairy products appear to be related to increased risk of metastatic prostate cancer. It appears that a proportion of the risk of metastatic PC is associated with red meat."[15,16]

It's not hard to find the biological plausibility of the meat-PC relationship. High in animal protein, saturated fat, cholesterol, and synthetic hormones, meat has it ALL.

Beef also has been shown to increase IGF-1 levels similar to dairy.[17] Beef fat also tends to absorb all of the chemicals that are used in modern beef production.[18] These dangerous chemicals bio-magnify (concentrate) in the fat of animals higher on the food chain because they are stored in body fat. It is estimated that up to 90% of the chemicals in our bodies come from eating animal products. Cooking beef, or any animal product for that matter, produces known cancer-causing metabolites called polycyclic aromatic hydrocarbons (PAC) and heterocyclic amines (HCA). Those beautiful grill marks on your barbeque fish, chicken, pork, and steak are the evidence of high-temperature creation of PAC's and

Chapter 33 – It's the Food

HCA's. For most of my life, meat of all types was grilled to the point of being burned, just the way I liked it. Ugh. And beef fat, in particular, has been shown to promote PC growth even compared to other fats.[19]

We have known for decades that high-fat diets increase the risk of most cancers.[20] High-fat foods are obviously high in calories, and we know excess calories promote cancer growth as well.[21]

Eggs

Everybody loves eggs. When Mindy and I lecture on foods to avoid, eggs always seem to be one of the most difficult foods for people to understand and give up. "What about the yolk?" "What about the white?" "What about the lower-left portion of the shell?" Anything to find justification to continue eating eggs. I ate probably at least two to three eggs a day for most of my life, believing the Egg Board ad that said, "Eggs are the perfect food." Well, they ain't. By a long shot. According to Dr. Neal Barnard, "There are only two problems with eggs: the yolk and the white."

An NIH funded study found that men consuming two-and-a-half eggs per week increased their risk for a deadly form of PC by 81% compared to those who ate just half an egg per week. The study followed 27,607 men who were part of the "Health Professionals Follow-up Study" from 1994 to 2008.[22]

But wait a minute! Aren't eggs, "the perfect food" as advertised by the Egg Board which is subsidized by our tax dollars and has an advertising budget of over $12 million? How can eggs be implicated in cancer development and progression? One culprit high on the list is choline which is an essential nutrient that is naturally present in some foods and is even available as a dietary supplement. It turns out that eggs have extremely high levels of choline which has been identified as a probable mechanistic link between egg and animal food consumption and PC.[23]

Eggs, along with chicken skin, are extremely high in choline in comparison to other animal foods. Choline is not only implicated in the development of PC, but it is also a leading suspect in more aggressive cancer. Choline, once absorbed by the gut, goes to the liver. The liver quickly oxidizes the substance and turns it into a substance called TMAO (Trimethylamine N-oxide) which is directly implicated in the progression of atherosclerosis as well as other chronic diseases.[24] The same Harvard researchers who discovered the cancer/choline connection also found a strong connection between choline consumption and more aggressive deadly PC. Eating two-and-a-half eggs per week may translate to an 81% increase risk of men dying from their PC.[25]

Chicken

The same Harvard study revealed that eating poultry and processed red meat increased the risk of aggressive cancer and early death. Men, with a high risk of recurrence, such as myself, are even more susceptible with a four-fold risk of recurrence or progression of PC compared to men who ate the least amount of eggs and chicken skin[26]. The Harvard researchers postulated that this may be due to the carcinogenic effect of heterocyclic amines and polycyclic aromatic hydrocarbons which, as mentioned previously, are the by-products of grilling any animal meat at high temperatures. According to the NIH, chicken is the largest source of cancer-causing heterocyclic amines in the American diet.[27]

And finally, the UCSF Cancer of the Prostate Strategic Urologic Research Endeavor (CaPSURE™) which is a longitudinal, observational study of 15,000 men with all stages of biopsy-proven prostate cancer found that post-diagnostic consumption of poultry with skin increases the risk of prostate cancer progression and cancer death.[28]

So there you have it with the chicken and the eggs. Why wouldn't every man diagnosed with PC give up chicken and eggs immediately? I did, and I know how difficult it is to change lifelong eating patterns without the proper tools. But it's not as difficult as you think, and the foods that will replace these disease-promoting animal foods are simply delicious! We can help you!

Fish and DHA/EPA

I am going to connect my analysis of fish with DHA/EPA because fish is the primary source of these fatty acids (EFA's) in the American diet. The ONLY two essential fatty acids (EFA's) are linoleic acid (an omega-6) and alpha-linolenic acid (a shorter-chain Omega-3). Essential fatty acids are those that cannot be synthesized by the body. EPA (Eicosapentaenoic acid) and DHA (Docosahexaenoic acid) can be manufactured by the body, albeit inefficiently, from alpha-linolenic acid.

Fish was a tough decision for me because I love fish and have eaten it my whole life with sushi being my favorite preparation. Like most Americans, I always assumed fish was a health-promoting choice of foods right up to... age 52 when I began reading and researching the relationship of PC with fish and DHA/EPA.

In 2011, Dr. Theodore Brasky, Ph.D., a researcher currently at the Ohio State University Comprehensive Cancer Center, conducted a nested case-control study of over 3500 participants from the Prostate Cancer Prevention Trial during 1994-2003. A defined sub-group is identified within a study and, for each individual, a specified number of matched controls is selected from among those in the cohort who have not developed the disease. The researchers examined the relationship between Omega-3 blood concentrations and PC. They discovered Docosahexaenoic acid (DHA) was positively associated with aggressive, high-grade prostate cancer![29] The researchers did not know if the DHA in the blood was from fish or a fish oil supplementation. OK, well-conducted, a large cohort, but just one study. Then, in the *Journal of the National Cancer Institute,* Dr. Brasky and his team published the results of another large study which duplicated their original findings in 2012. The

Selenium and Vitamin E Cancer Prevention Trial (SELECT) showed that DHA, which is the primary fat of fish and the main active component in fish oil tablets, significantly increased the risk of high-grade (Gleason 8 and above) prostate cancer.[30,31]

That same year, an Italian group of researchers reported conclusive negative findings on supplemental DHA's ability to decrease heart attacks or delay heart disease progression,[32] which was DHA's major claim to fame by the supplement industry to begin with.

As I mentioned earlier, we don't know if the high DHA levels in these men came from eating fish or taking supplements. It looks to me like fish oil (DHA/EPA) supplements fail across the board, but what about just eating fish? Specifically, fish consumption and prostate cancer risk have been analyzed by many scientists, and the results are, well, inconclusive. A Swedish cohort of 6,272 men found that those who consumed no fish had a 2 to 3-fold increase in the risk of developing PC compared to those who consumed large amounts of fish.[33] And a prospective cohort study from the "Physicians' Health Study" found fish consumption was not related to PC risk but was protective of PC death.[34]

However, the Fred Hutchinson Cancer Center team that found the link between aggressive PC and DHA blood levels outlined above have come to a different conclusion: "This large prospective investigation of inflammation-associated phospholipid fatty acids and prostate cancer risk found no support that n-3 fatty acids (DHA/EPA) decrease prostate cancer risk. Our findings are disconcerting as they suggest that n-3 fatty acids, considered beneficial for coronary artery disease prevention, may increase high-grade prostate cancer."

Several additional papers have been published that support a weak link with DHA/EPA and an increased risk of PC including "the most extensive systematic review to assess the effects of polyunsaturated fatty acids" (PUFAs). This review, published in the *British Medical Journal* (BMJ) included 47 long-term RCT's randomizing 108k participants, and found increasing total PUFA may very slightly increase cancer risk.[35]

I could not find a specific recommendation one way or the other for fish consumption on the Fred Hutch website (https://www.fredhutch.org/), but the organization makes a strong recommendation to avoid DHA/EPA supplements[36] based on both the SELECT study results as well as the similar finding from the seven-year Prostate Cancer Prevention Trial, a randomized, placebo-controlled trial that evaluated the effect of finasteride on prostate cancer risk[37] during 1994-2003, concluding: "The consistency of these findings suggests that these fatty acids are involved in prostate tumorigenesis, and recommendations to increase long-chain Omega-3 fatty acid intake, in particular through supplementation, should consider its potential risks."

I corresponded with Dr. Brasky, and he made an important point "that there is far less research on dietary fats and fatty acids among men already diagnosed with prostate cancer. I wouldn't necessarily equate your conclusions from my research on prostate cancer risk among men without prostate cancer with progression among men diagnosed with prostate cancer. These are different things."

What are us guys with recurrent PC supposed to do? The saturated fat and animal protein link with PC discussed previously align with the Fred Hutch Cancer Center outcomes: "Our findings clearly show decreased risk for late-stage disease in men with diets that are low in fat and moderate in calcium, perhaps because of these diets slow progression of prostate cancer into a more aggressive disease."

Salmon and shellfish have significantly higher cholesterol and saturated fat in comparison to other seafoods. And the higher on the food chain, the higher the concentration of environmental chemicals in the ocean ecosystem. This bio-magnification occurs because these chemicals are stored in body fat, just like land animals. So, when the fish eat other fish with chemical contamination, they become concentrated in the fish's fatty tissues. After we eat the fish fat (or any animal fat for that matter), most of these chemicals are transferred to our own fat tissues. As discussed previously, most of the man-made chemicals in our bodies come from eating meat, poultry, fish, and dairy products.[38] Simply removing animal products from your diet will eliminate these chemicals over time, and that's exactly what I have done.

The majority of fish available in the US is now factory farmed.[39] These industrialized factory-produced fish have higher levels of the inflammation-promoting Omega-6 fats, saturated fat, and cholesterol, but lower amounts of the supposedly health-promoting DHA/EPA long-chain Omega-3 fatty acids that we were trying to get in the first place![40]

The supplement industry also advertises that fish oil supposedly improves cognitive health. The National Institute of Health (NIH) completed one of the largest and longest clinical trials of Omega-3 fatty acids and brain health with 4000 patients which were followed over a five-year period. The study was published in the *Journal of the American Medical Association* in 2015. Bottom line: Even after five years, the NIH found that Omega-3 supplements did not slow cognitive decline in older persons.[41]

This is the current status of fishing and eating fish on the planet: More than 80% of the fish oil being produced is now being fed to farmed fish in an attempt to increase DHA/EPA levels in the fish meat itself! This is absolutely CRAZY based on the research to date.

I made a specific point to ask Dr. Michael Greger, Dr. T. Colin Campbell, Dr. Michael Klaper, and Dr. Neal Barnard about the DHA/EPA research situation and the recommendation by some PC organizations to consume fish in light of the Fred Hutch research showing higher levels of DHA / EPA in the blood being associated with more aggressive PC.

~ ~ ~

Chapter 33 – It's the Food

Expert Analysis—Dr. Michael Greger

I'm surprised fish is recommended. It's possible they're recommending fish in hopes it'll be eaten instead of red meat. If your choice is between olive oil and butter, olive oil is better, and if your choice is between a steak and fish, then fish is better. They may be assuming men wouldn't actually go that next step and actually eat only plant-based diets which is a patronizing attitude. We know you're not gonna do what you really need to do, so we're going to give you these half measures, which are achievable, but we're talking about cancer here.

You want every single possible tweak and technique to try to slow progression as much as possible. And so that's why it shouldn't be about compromise, it should be very clear this is the ideal diet. And then, look, if you can't do that, here are some half measures. Right, okay, well, at least let's get rid of processed meat. At least you gotta cut dairy out. At least do this X, Y, and Z. It should be made very clear: Here's the ideal diet, and if you want the odds on your side, this is the way you have to go.

A low-fat whole-food, plant-based diet is Dr. Greger's recommendation without any fish on the plate based on his latest research.

Dr. T. Colin Campbell

Dr. Campbell discusses what has lead up to the current situation:

> With fish, there's this bit of trade-off. A lot of the fish in the ocean are contaminated with hydrocarbons, for example, and they don't go away, there they are. They accumulate, and that's not good. But then there's some deep-water, more pristine kinds of fish that don't accumulate in quite the same way, and we think they should be okay. They do have Omega-3 fats, which is anti-inflammatory. I'm just trying to tell it as the story unfolded.
>
> But it turns out that the protein in fish, regardless of what kind it is, operates about the same way as the protein in land animals. They both tend to increase blood pressure. They both do some other things that are all worse. I don't see fish protein and what goes with it to be much different from land animals. That's number one.

Chapter 33 – It's the Food

Number two, when we're eating fish, just like when we're eating land animals, we're displacing some of the good stuff, including the antioxidant carbohydrates from plants. So, I think fish is in the same category as land animals, but I'm open to others' analyses.

The Omega-3 story is falling apart. Omega-6 and Omega-3 are the two fats that pair against each other in the body. And the body knows how to manipulate them. Omega-6 is pro-inflammatory and contributes to heart disease. At a scientific level, the body needs some Omega-6. That's without a doubt. Omega-6 comes in because the body's using the balance of Omega-6 to Omega-3 to fight foreign organisms and infectious diseases. So they have a role to play by the ratio of one to the other, and the best ratio, according to various kinds of data, is 2:1 or 3:1 of Omega-6 to Omega-3. Presently, in the American diet, it runs around 15:1, which is ridiculous. We are getting a lot of Omega-6 coming from all of the oils we eat, and it leaves most of us in a pro-inflammatory state.

Now, in this pro-inflammatory circumstance, and you give them Omega-3, you can see something in the short run, and it looks pretty good, which is not surprising, because you're dumping in some Omega-3 to counter some of that Omega-6. But at the end of the day, after watching a number of studies being done, the Omega-3 supplements don't work either, even though we might see some benefits of overall indication early on.

Dr. Neal Barnard

There's been some really puzzling literature that I don't understand yet on Omega-3. A lot of men take fish oil hoping to not have a heart attack, and it turns out it doesn't work very well or at all for staving off a heart attack. However, researchers started looking at prostate cancer and found that men taking fish oil had more prostate cancer which seemed like a fluke. And one or two studies didn't show the same connection, so maybe it really was a fluke. But then more and more researchers have been looking at this, and for whatever reason, guys who take Omega-3s as supplements are at higher risk of prostate cancer compared to other men, and we don't know why.

Chapter 33 – It's the Food

Algae-based vegan supplements have not been looked at separately, and I think that's just because nobody was taking it as it's a new product. It was fish oil that was really under scrutiny, and what's been troubling is, nobody knows why. First of all, it may not be real. It's just that so many studies are showing that the men who take this have more prostate cancer, and I take it seriously. Nobody could figure out why or what's the mechanism. Another issue is that some people will say, "Well, maybe Omega-3s, although they're not so good for your heart, maybe they'll reduce Alzheimer's risk." Possible, I don't know. My advice is that if a person is going to take Omega supplements, you can get tested and see if your Omega-3 blood level is low. I'm not saying you have to take them at all, but if a person is going to, I would suggest getting tested first. If you're not low, why are you bothering? And you have to decide, okay, is my fear of Alzheimer's bigger than my fear of prostate cancer, or whatever. And unfortunately, we're in one of these situations where science just doesn't have the answers people want. We just don't. And so, in that ambiguity, people have to make choices based

> on the evidence that they have. And if prostate cancer looms up as a threat in a person's life, it's pretty hard to avoid making the life choices that minimize your risk of progression, and those are probably the very same things that contributed to its development in the first place. So I would say if a person is going to take a fish oil or DHA/EPA supplement, get tested first. It's not for me to tell men or women what to do. Here's what we know, and based on that, people have to make their own choices."

Dr. Michael Klaper

> I would prefer to see you get your Omega-3's from nuts like walnuts, flax seeds, and leafy green vegetables until the DHA / EPA situation gets sorted out.

There is no research indicating that adding fish to a healthy diet increases health even more. The "Adventist II Health Study" also demonstrated that fish eaters are at a higher risk of diabetes and have a higher body mass index compared to plant eaters.[42] We know we want to minimize body fat when fighting PC! And the final nail in the "fish" coffin for me is: The United Nations has declared "fishing to be a net economic loss to the world".[43] Humans are stripping the oceans of natural wild fish.

Chapter 33 – It's the Food

The *European Journal of Clinical Nutrition* investigated fish consumption in Mediterranean diets and came to the following conclusion: "Fish consumption is not positively correlated with heart disease mortality. That suggests that dietary factors other than fish, such as the lower meat consumption associated to the higher fish intake or other differences of lifestyle have come into play, helping to explain the healthy nature of the Mediterranean diet."[44]

My decision: I love fish, but it's off the menu for me. No fish, no fish oil, and no vegan DHA supplements. The research to date does not support any of it in my opinion. By the way, I don't miss fish at ALL, and you won't either if you take the time to explore all the flavors the plant kingdom has to offer.

In order to assure adequate Omega-3 consumption, I eat two tablespoons of fresh ground flax on my boiled breakfast cereal (whole grain groats *which* are whole grains that include the cereal germ and fiber-rich bran portion of the grain, as well as the endosperm) in the morning. Boiled whole grains have been consumed since recorded history and is usually referred to as "congee." Fresh ground flax seeds have the highest concentration of the parent Omega-3 fatty acid, which is known as alpha-linolenic acid (ALA). ALA is the only essential Omega-3 fatty acid required from the diet with walnuts and flax seeds having the highest concentration. ALA can then be converted to the longer-chain Omega-3 fatty (EPA, DHA) acids by the body.

Supplements

I am not a big fan of supplements for supporting prostate cancer healing or health in general. The balance of government-funded independent research has demonstrated that the vast majority of supplements are either ineffective and, in some cases, outright dangerous. Case in point: DHA/EPA supplements covered in the previous chapter with fish.

There have been several large, randomized trials that have investigated the use of dietary supplements and the risk of various cancers, including prostate. All demonstrated either no effect or, even more concerning—they have shown significantly increased risk.

According to Alan Kristal, Dr.P.H. (https://www.fredhutch.org/en/news/center-news/2019/03/kristal-obit-cancer-prevention.html), Associate Director of the Hutchinson Center's Cancer Prevention Program and a national expert in prostate cancer prevention, "The more we look at the effects of taking supplements, the more hazardous they appear when it comes to cancer risk." He cites that the "Selenium and Vitamin E Cancer Prevention Trial" (SELECT), the largest prostate cancer prevention study to date, was stopped early because it found neither selenium nor vitamin E supplements, alone or combined, reduced the risk of prostate cancer. Additionally, A SELECT follow-up study published recently in JAMA found that vitamin E actually increased the risk of prostate cancer among

Chapter 33 – It's the Food

healthy men. The study involved nearly 35,000 men in the U.S., Canada, and Puerto Rico.

What has become clear is that isolating specific nutrients, antioxidants, and vitamins, and putting them in a pill does not have the same effect as consuming whole plants. Nature did not design our bodies to consume, metabolize, and utilize isolated nutrients in high dosages. The research to date suggests the optimum way to fuel your body with antioxidants, vitamins, and minerals is to get them through food in the form of seeds, nuts, vegetables, grains, legumes, and fruit. That's what I do. The $60 million supplement industry is the poster child of reductionist science at its worst: "Let's find the magic component of an apple, or any other healthy food, isolate it in a lab, and put a lot of it in a pill and sell it to unassuming consumers without sufficient research."

The U.S. Preventive Services Task Force is an independent panel of experts in primary care and prevention that systematically reviews the evidence of the effectiveness of dietary supplements and develops recommendations for clinical preventive services. These reviews are published as U.S. Preventive Services Task Force (USPSTF) recommendations on the Task Force website (https://www.uspreventiveservicestaskforce.org/) and in a peer-reviewed journal. In 2012, based on all evidence to date, the USPSTF DOES NOT recommend the use of ANY multivitamins or herbal supplements. They also go so far as to advise consumers NOT to take beta-carotene or vitamin E.[45]

Dr. Mark Moyad (https://pcri.org/mark-moyad) is Director of Preventive/Complementary and Alternative Medicine at the University of Michigan Medical Center in the Department of Urology. *Prevention Magazine* has called Dr. Mark Moyad "Arguably, the world's leading medical expert on dietary supplements." He has published *The Supplement Handbook: A Trusted Expert's Guide to What Works & What's Worthless for More Than 100 Conditions,* which outlines the best research to date and his recommendations on specific supplements for specific concerns. It is well researched and useful when evaluating supplements. Dr. Moyad has done a lot of specific research into supplements for prostate cancer as well as for the PCRI (Prostate Cancer Research Institute). Dr. Michael Greger also has extensive video and written research summaries on supplements available on his website and in his books.

I avoid doctors and medical professionals that sell supplements and/or have them on display in their office. To me, this represents someone who is more interested in selling pills for profit than focusing on patient needs. In my opinion, treating physicians should NOT be selling supplements, period.

I stick with a simple 250 mg of vitamin B12 as a sublingual twice a week along with 1000 micrograms of D3 a few times a week in the winter if I'm not out in the sun much. I try to get at least 15 minutes of total skin sun exposure most days. Both my D3 and my B12 levels are in the healthy range, and I don't worry about them. I wish I could say that about my PSA!

Chapter 33 – It's the Food

Summary

1. The single most important risk factor identified for prostate cancer is an increased blood level of IGF-1.
2. Eggs, dairy, and animal foods, in general, have been identified as the most likely food suspects with the diet and prostate cancer connection.
3. Fish is not required in the human diet. DHA, which is the primary fat of fish and the main active component in fish oil tablets, significantly increases the risk of high-grade prostate cancer.

CHAPTER 34
PLANT OILS—THE FOOD FAT CONNECTION

Olive oil is the table salt of fats.

— Dr. Michael Greger

Plant oils such as olive oil, MCT (medium-chain triglycerides) oil, and avocado oil are also concerns for PC patients. Processed plant oils are the foundation of almost every meal prepared in any restaurant around the world. Processed plant oils are snuck into almost ALL packaged foods and in processed foods as well. I'll make this easy: The balance of recent research has made it is very clear that pure, isolated vegetable fats in the form of oil suppress the immune system and artery function. Just like animal fats, these isolated fats can encourage cancer growth. High-fat diets (both animal and vegetable) tend to be high in chemical contaminants and raise hormone levels, including testosterone.[1] I am pretty sure my goal is NOT to raise my testosterone!

Comparisons of the fat intake in scores of different countries show that populations with the highest per capita fat consumption have the highest breast cancer mortality.[2] However, Dr. Walter Willet of Harvard found no relationship between dietary fat and breast cancer incidence with the 90,000 participants in the "Nurses' Health Study."[3] The exceedingly small differences in the fat intake of the population investigated in the NHS (between 32% and 44% of total calories), is most likely why this massive study showed no association. A true low-fat diet is less than 15% of calories from fat! There has simply been no long-term study comparing a true low-fat diet (less than 15% of calories from fat) to the standard American diet of 30-45% of calories from fat. "The Nurses' Health Study" was comparing two high-fat diets to one another. Dr. Campbell describes the "Nurses' Health Study" as "an investigation of carnivorous nurses."

I also believe the NHS is a great example for those of us trying to improve our cancer outcomes, and this is reflected in Dr. Barnard's statement: "Small changes, small results. Drastic changes, drastic results." I (we) want drastic results!

According to Dr. John McDougall, "Fats of all kinds, including vegetable fats and 'health-food' olive and flaxseed oils, are easily oxidized into highly reactive molecules which trigger a host of cancer-causing processes, including damaging our DNA. Fortunately, these reactions are stopped by antioxidants, such as vitamin E, lycopene (found in red-pigmented plants), and selenium, all found in plant foods. Thus, fats of all kinds may also influence cancer development by a variety of mechanisms."

On Dr. McDougall's website, he cites a 2001 study out of Denmark in which men with PC on a 34-day low-fat diet (20% fat, which is still high in my opinion) supplemented with an ounce of flaxseeds daily decreased total serum cholesterol, testosterone, and free androgen. Additionally, PSA levels went down, not up, and cancer growth at the microscopic level went down. All markers continued to improve the longer they were on the diet.[4]

Turning point! Or maybe "tweaking" point:

> After converting to a plant-based diet in 2011, both Mindy and I continued to consume a lot of olive oil. We also did not pay much attention to the amount of added plant oils, such as soy oil, in processed foods, and we definitely did not even think about all the oil in restaurant foods. Then in 2015, we attended one of Dr. McDougall's weekend retreats in Santa Rosa, CA. Big surprise: Across the board, the experts at this summit (Dr. John McDougal, Dr. Caldwell Esselstyn, Dr. T. Colin Campbell) all strongly recommended eliminating ALL oils from our diets. All oils, including olive oil, raise triglycerides (fat in the blood) and as a result, decrease flow-mediated dilation

of our blood vessels, making them less pliable.[5]

It appears that the well-studied health benefits of the Mediterranean diet may be due to the abundance of minimally processed plant foods IN SPITE OF THE OLIVE OIL. Just remember: All oil, including olive oil, is 100% processed fat, with the vast majority of the nutrients and all the fiber being removed during processing. And as Dr. McDougall likes to point out: "The fat you eat is the fat you wear."

Since attending that conference, we have done our best to eliminate all added oils to our diets. Every single one of our onedaytowellness.org video recipes is made without added oil. It's very easy once you get the hang of it. Try it yourself! Commit to going a full week without eating any added oil to your food. You discover two things:

1. It's almost impossible to eat at a restaurant.
2. After adjusting to no added oil in your food, you will immediately taste (with an oily displeasure), the slippery goop and want to spit it out of your mouth. This is how quickly your taste buds and your gut will adapt to a no-oil diet if you simply give them a chance.

Here is what I have learned for myself: Change your diet, change your life. That's the beautiful thing about evidence-based nutritional intervention and PC: You can still do it along with whatever treatment you and your oncologist decide is the best approach. Moving towards a more plant-based diet only has positive side effects. Traditional treatment, not so much.

Summary

1. "Free fats," including canola, soy, olive oil, and flaxseed oil are not health foods.
2. All oil, including olive oil, is 100% processed fat, with the vast majority of the nutrients and all the fiber being removed during processing.
3. Commit to giving up oil for just one week and then see how you feel.

CHAPTER 35
WHAT DO I EAT?

Ask not what you can do for your country. Ask what's for lunch.

— Orson Welles

I have spent a fair number of pages discussing the evidence behind what we now know is disease-promoting food, which is basically what I ate my whole life without even realizing it. Now let's take a quick tour of plant-based foods and the health they can create.

First of all, vegan diets are safe and effective for prostate cancer patients.[1] Even the Academy of Nutrition and Dietetics (AND), the organization that registers dieticians and has long been criticized for their cozy relationship with the beef, egg, dairy, chicken, and junk food industries (over the past five years, AND's most loyal partners have been Aramark, Coca-Cola, and the National Dairy Council along with junk food producers PepsiCo, Kellogg, Mars, and General Mills) has stated that vegan and plant-based diets are safe and effective.[2]

Protein

All protein originates from the plant kingdom. The largest mammals on the planet are vegan: Cows eat grass and get all the protein they need. Elephants eat grass, small plants, twigs, and tree bark to acquire protein. Gorillas eat leaves and fruit to obtain all the protein they need. The best source of protein for humans comes from plants.

Expert Opinion / Dr. Alan Goldhamer

> In addition to parasites, bacterial infestation, toxic poisons, carcinogenic agents, and free radicals, animal products all suffer from the problem of biological concentration. All animal products are completely devoid of fiber and are extremely high in protein, and in spite of what millions of dollars of meat and dairy industry advertising would have you believe, it is excess, not inadequate protein, that is the threat to health. Excess protein intake has been strongly implicated as a causal agent in many disease processes including kidney disease, various forms of cancer, osteoporosis, and a host of autoimmune and hypersensitivity disease processes.
>
> It is ironic that the chief argument used to promote the use of animal products—

that is, the purported need for large quantities of protein—is the greatest reason for avoiding them.

A diet of sufficient caloric intake derived from fresh fruits and vegetables with the variable addition of nuts, whole grains, and legumes will provide an optimum intake of protein and other nutrients, 30-70 grams per day, depending upon the particular foods eaten.

The World Health Organization (WHO) recommends 50 grams of protein a day FROM PLANT SOURCES.[3] The average American eats in excess of 100 grams of protein per day, primarily from animal sources.[4] You get all the protein you need, and in the best form, from plants. There is no need to worry about combining foods either. Simply eating a varied and colorful WFPB diet with plenty of whole grains will ensure you get all essential nutrients, including complete protein.

Phytochemicals

Only plants produce phytochemicals (plant-based chemicals). You will never receive the cancer-fighting powers of phytochemicals if you don't EAT THEM. Specifically, one group of phytochemicals, isoflavones, was discovered to inhibit the growth of prostate cancer in mice.[5]

Minimally processed soy foods such as edamame, tofu, and tempeh have high levels of isoflavones in comparison to other plant foods. Do not believe what you hear from the soy doubters! Go to the research! Several large and long-term cohort studies have consistently demonstrated that soy consumption decreases both the risk of breast cancer and the risk of recurrence.[6,7,8,9] According to the American Institute of Cancer Research, "Population studies don't link soy consumption with increased risk of any cancer, and limited evidence shows either no effect or decreased risk of prostate cancer. Observational studies also link moderate soy consumption (one to two servings a day) with lower breast cancer risk in Asia, where soy foods are commonly consumed throughout life." Don't freak out about soy! Replacing an eight-ounce steak with a giant piece of tofu is not a good idea. Use tofu as a condiment, not the main dish. We have several organic tofu and tempeh recipes on our recipes at onedaytowellness.org.

Additional phytochemicals include beta carotene found in orange pumpkins, sweet potatoes, and carrots. Lycopene is the red pigment found in cooked tomato products, watermelon, and red bell peppers. Anthocyanidins give blueberries and blackberries their dark blue pigment. There are thousands of phytochemicals that include antioxidants such as vitamin C in every plant food, including grains such as barley, rye, wheat, and kamut, to name just a few (more on whole grains later). Phytochemicals have been discovered to have many

Chapter 35 – What Do I Eat?

disease-fighting compounds that strengthen our immune system, repel viral attacks in our bodies, and mitigate cancer initiation and progression.

I consider ALL whole plant foods to be "superfoods." You cannot expect including a few "superfoods" to counteract a bad diet. All fruits, legumes, grains, and vegetables are good for you. Just make sure that they are making up the majority of your diet. If you hear or read about a "superfood," in all likelihood, there is a sales pitch coming for a new supplement to add to your budget and to your urine. Save the money and just eat plants!

Fiber

The World Health Organization recommends getting between 25 to 30 grams of fiber a day in the diet. Here in the US, less than 3% of the population even comes close! According to the USDA, the average American eats less than 16 grams per day.[10] It's simply ridiculous, especially with the emerging research of the additional benefit of lots of fiber in our diet. It is the body's "prebiotic," which means the preferred food of our healthy gut bacteria. When our healthy gut bacteria consumes undigestible soluble fiber, it is fermented into a host of health-promoting chemicals and compounds such as the short-chain fatty acid butyrate. Recent research has discovered butyrate to be one of the most powerful health-promoting substances in our body that helps to accelerate apoptosis (cell death), decrease tumor invasiveness, and blunting cancer cell proliferation.[11] So the next time someone asks you, "You don't eat meat, where do you get your protein?" Ask them in return, "You choose meat over fruit and veggies? Where do you get your fiber?"

Summary

1. A WFPB diet provides just the right amount of protein required by humans—50 grams a day. The average American eats more than 100 grams of protein per day, primarily from animal sources. Stop worrying about protein.
2. Phytochemicals (only found in plant food) have been discovered to have many cancer-fighting compounds which strengthen our immune system, repel viral attacks in our bodies, and mitigate cancer initiation and progression.
3. Focus on getting more fiber in your diet in the form of grains, beans, and leafy veggies.

CHAPTER 36
TURNING POINTS—INTERMITTENT FASTING AND INTACT GRAINS

Fasting is the greatest remedy—the physician within.

— Philippus Paracelsus
one of the three fathers
of Western medicine

Intermittent Fasting

I'll briefly discuss the latest research on fasting and cancer, but that's straightforward. First, my personal perspective: Fasting is AWESOME. When I complete (I did not say "during") a prolonged water-only fast, which for me is three to five days every month, I feel like a newer, younger, higher energy person. For me personally, it FEELS like the fountain of youth! The only challenge is actually doing it. Fasting is difficult, but achievable and doable. I have some great tips, but first, the research.

As you may recall, I first became aware of fasting as a tool to battle cancer while Mindy and I were on a self-guided bike tour of Tuscany in the spring of 2017. I had purchased the book, *The Pleasure Trap*, by Dr. Douglas Lisle and Dr. Alan Goldhamer, founders of the TrueNorth Health Center, and I read it at the end of each exhausting day of biking through the rolling hills of Northern Italy. Dr. Goldhamer and his team at the TrueNorth Health Center routinely bring severely chronically ill individuals back to health using the ancient technique of medical supervised water-only fasting. TrueNorth is the leading research facility for water-only fasting, and I wanted to give it a go. What really piqued my interest was a case study documented by Dr. Goldhamer of a woman with Stage 4 lymphoma whose lesions disappeared after 45 days of water-only fasting at their clinic.[1] Forty-five days? Really? As I read through the history and the documented power of fasting to bring people off of diabetic, blood pressure, triglyceride, and thyroid medication, to name just a few, I was convinced. What is the downside? From a medical perspective, there really isn't any for someone like me who is highly motivated to try nutritional therapy, including water-only fasting, to slow the growth of PC in my body. Here is a quick summary on what's happening with fasting and cancer:

Fasting and caloric restriction has been proven to increase life span in yeast, fruit flies, and rats.[2] Seeing the same effects of caloric restriction across many different types of living tissues gives credence to the strong possibility that it will have the same effects in

Chapter 36 – Turning Points—Intermittent Fasting...

humans. But, as Doctor Greger says, "You've got to put it to the test." Research on humans is still in its infancy, but there are several programs and studies underway looking at human caloric restriction. We do know that many of the molecular pathways that are altered with calorie restriction are also known to be altered in cancer. Manipulating these pathways using fasting or caloric restriction can render cancer cells more susceptible to standard cytotoxic treatment with radiation and chemotherapy. *The Oncologist Magazine* reported on research from the Chicago Medical School which showed that restricting calories just by 15% in patients having radiotherapy produced better results and fewer side effects compared to a control group that had only radio therapy.[3] From there, it was postulated the same might be true of chemotherapy and calorie restriction. Dr. Valter Longo and his team of researchers at USC have demonstrated fasting coupled with chemo improves outcomes in mice with cancer.4 For all cancers tested, fasting combined with chemotherapy improved survival, slowed tumor growth, and/or limited the spread of tumors in all the cancers tested in mice. Longo stated that fasting started a "cascade of events" that led to the creation of damaging free radical molecules, which broke down the cancer cells' own DNA and caused their destruction.

The USC team also completed a small study with ten older cancer patients who took on short-term fasting prior to and after each chemo session. All of these patients reported improved ability to withstand the chemo and improved mitigation of side-effects such as nausea and fatigue.

According to Longo, fasting actually stopped cancer cells from producing "protection proteins" from their mutated genes, while healthy cells made more of them. This causes healthy cells to stop dividing and become less vulnerable to chemotherapy resulting in lowered side-effects. Some combinations of fasting and chemotherapy actually made tumors disappear! The result: Fasting improves chemo efficacy as well as blunting the side effects.

Longo's team also discovered that caloric restriction deprives cancer cells of glucose, so it looks like multiple synergistic activities are at work here.

A 2019 study investigating mice with implanted breast cancer, melanoma, or glioma cells, showed that short-term fasting ALONE delayed tumor growth to the same extent as treatment with the chemo drug cyclophosphamide![5]

Test results on rodents usually do not translate to people. Multiple cancer centers around the world are working on two large human clinical trials investigating the side-effects reduction phenomenon of fasting as well as improving chemo efficacy. Regarding PC, the National Institute of Health is close to completion of a trial looking at fasting in patients with advanced metastatic, castration-resistant, PC.[6]

This is a randomized trial of 60 men, investigating both fasting for chemotherapy and its efficacy. As of the writing of this book, the results have not been released. You can check the clinicaltrials.gov website (https://clinicaltrials.gov/) for updates.

But hold on! Even with the known benefits of fasting coupled with chemotherapy, according to a USC poll, 70% of cancer patients would refuse a water-only fasting regime if offered. All I can say is, WOW! Come on guys; we can do better than this! We are dealing with cancer here, not the flu (or Covid19 for that matter). Bite the bullet and start the meaningful journey of changing your habits and behaviors to help you STAY ALIVE.

Don't plan on Big Pharma funding any of these research studies. How much money is there in telling people not to eat? However, Big Pharma WILL NOT LIKE the idea of using fasting to REDUCE drug use. Some are now investigating if fasting could allow patients to use EVEN MORE DRUGS.

Turning Point or Tweaking POINT

Whole Intact Grains

During my discussion with Dr. Gordon Saxe regarding his research at UCSD, I had another "turning point" in my nutritional journey to fight PC. Dr. Saxe relayed to me the story of Dr. Tony Sattilaro, former president of Methodist Hospital in Philadelphia.

In 1978, Dr. Sattilaro found out he had prostate cancer that had metastasized to his skull, shoulder, and backbone, and was given about one year to live. Driving home one day, he picked up a few hitchhikers. During the drive, Dr. Sattilaro revealed to his passengers his situation and prognosis. One of the hitchhikers commented, "You don't have to die, Dr. S; you can cure your cancer."

Dr. S, who had been an MD for 25 years and worked with some of the best cancer specialists in the world, just rolled his eyes but kept listening. His new friend convinced Dr. S. to visit a foundation in Philadelphia that advocated a macrobiotic diet approach to cancer and taught cooking classes. The diet consisted of 50% cooked whole grains including wheat, barley, brown rice, and millet, plus 25% vegetables, 15% beans and sea vegetables, along with nuts and seeds. Essentially, a low-fat, starch-rich, whole-food, plant-based diet. The entire diet was a complete departure of Dr. S's lifelong consumption of meat, dairy, eggs, and processed foods. He initially thought it was just a bunch of mumbo jumbo, but he quickly came to the conclusion, "What do I have to lose?" and dove into the cooking classes and the new diet. Within two weeks, Dr. S's pain from the metastasis was GONE. That's right; metastatic prostate cancer bone pain had simply resolved. In September of 1979, 15 months after beginning his new diet, a bone scan revealed his body and his bones to be free of cancer. Dr. Sattilaro stated, "It was a miracle," and wrote a book about his experience entitled *Recalled by Life* and then another called *Living Well Naturally.*

Chapter 36 – Turning Points—Intermittent Fasting...

Unfortunately, in the late 1980s, Dr. Sattilaro drifted off the diet, and his cancer returned, and he passed in 1989. Damn! I wanted a better ending! But even though Dr. S eventually succumbed to his PC, he did prove to himself that the largest effect he could elicit on his cancer was not years of drugs and procedures (he had them all), but a simple change from a disease-promoting diet to a health-promoting one.

The theme and idea of using basic minimally processed cooked grains to treat PC kept coming up in Dr. Saxe's and my discussion.

~ ~ ~

Expert Analysis—Dr. Gordon Saxe

> Intact kernel whole grains are very different than refined grain products. They're like opposite ends of the spectrum in terms of harmful or healing. When grains are in the intact kernel form, the food is vital and alive. It could germinate and grow a new plant. Cut that whole oat into steel-cut oats, and it may look pretty healthy, but it has been devitalized and can no longer germinate, and it begins to oxidize when you breach the bran layer, losing its nutrient composition quite rapidly.
>
> Also, when you grind that 100% whole grain, like whole wheat berry, into 100%

whole wheat flour, you've now taken that starch, the endosperm on the inside, and you've magnified its surface area like 1000-fold, which means the body can take it up and convert it to glucose much more rapidly. The glycemic response to the devitalized flower is much greater than to the intact kernel whole grain. This translates into spiking blood sugar and a resulting higher insulin anemic response. More insulin has to be made to relieve that spike and push sugar into cells. As long as that's your pattern, then you can't lose weight as readily, and the insulin is essentially like a headwind. You can't break down the fat from the cells back into component parts. So, there's a benefit to intact kernel whole grains as your complex carb source. But there's yet another advantage. Intact kernel whole grain holds on to the starch, and it resists digestion in the upper GI tract, and large particles make it down to the lower GI tract. In the large intestine, resistant starch ferments and becomes the basic food source for healthy microbes in the gut. Those microbes then produce their own ketone bodies in the form of butyrate and butyric acid, which are anti-inflammatory, anti-cancer properties in the gut, and get into the bloodstream.

Chapter 36 – Turning Points—Intermittent Fasting...

So, a different way of going into a ketonic state is the combination of intact kernel whole-grain-based, whole food plant-based nutrition, coupled with intermittent fasting. Now, instead of an animal food that comes with all the saturated fat, you're now getting plant-based fats from an intact whole grain kernel, which is beneficial because your gut bacteria are getting coupled with intermittent cannibalization of your own fat stores, which break down senescent (old) cells. And what's not to like about that? I feel like one mission I have is to share with vegans the importance of intact kernel whole grains properly prepared.

Congee is the traditional term for boiled, intact whole grains. It could be brown rice, whole barley, whole oats, millet, Job's tears, amaranth, teff, or any number of intact kernel whole grains. It's just a porridge made from an intact kernel, whole grain, and water in proportion to the grain, slow cooked. It's made into a kind of a goopy, mucilaginous, fully cooked porridge, which is easy for somebody with weakened power of digestion to absorb, process, and eliminate the waste. It's a great way to provide nutrition to somebody who's weak and depleted. And it's a great way to help alleviate digestive ailments like constipation and/or diarrhea in people whose bowels aren't moving and can't eliminate waste properly. Traditionally, it was used as a first food in Chinese medicine, including Ayurveda healing systems around the world. Hippocrates used it as one of his first primary healing approaches. He made congee out of whole barley and called it Tizann. It's been used in Turkey where it's called Laba. In Korea, they call it Juk. In Japan, they call it Okayu.

These have always been healing approaches, not just healing for an individual, but for humanity. If we are going to feed nine or ten billion people, one of the most efficient ways to do it is with intact kernel whole grains.

Since my discussion with Dr. Saxe, Mindy and I have transitioned to eating ALL of our whole grains, including kamut, farrow, oat, buckwheat, rye, and barley, in the intact, boiled form. Up to this point, we always ate oatmeal for breakfast, but now we have some derivative of congee. It varies day to day, but since the transition, I have noticed:

1. I love the varied grains, flavor, and texture.
2. I stay full much longer than with oatmeal.

3. We now prepare whole cooked grains concoctions instead of rice for ALL of our meals. It's fun, and the new flavors and textures are fantastic.

What's the downside of giving congee or boiled intact whole grains a try? NONE whatsoever. DON'T LEAVE MONEY ON THE TABLE!

Dr. John McDougall has been promoting a low-fat vegan starch-based diet for healing AND weight loss for decades. He outlines the details of his lifelong eating approach in his book, *The Starch Solution,* as approximately 70% starch (in the form of whole foods such as potatoes, intact grains, and legumes), 20% vegetables, and 10% fruits. High-fat plant-based foods like avocado, nuts, and seeds are kept to a strict minimum if consumed at all. No oil. Soy protein like tofu and tempeh are also kept to a minimum, though they're not as strictly limited as dietary fat. Starches in the form of whole intact grains, potatoes, and legumes are naturally filling foods that keep me satiated. My eating strategy basically is to follow Dr. McDougall's suggestions, but I do include some nuts and avocados in my diet. I do my best to avoid all added oils as well, which can prove very challenging, especially if you decide to leave your house!

Summary

1. Fasting can be a powerful tool in your PC battle on multiple fronts: slowing the growth

of cancer, increasing chemotherapy efficacy, and mitigation of side-effects such as nausea and fatigue.
2. Eat intact grains. They have the least amount of processing and the most nutrition compared to oatmeal, etc. And they taste fantastic!
3. The combination of intact kernel whole-grains as part of your whole food plant-based nutrition, coupled with intermittent fasting, may be the most powerful natural tools you have to fight PC.

CHAPTER 37
GOING FORWARD

If you don't focus on the future generation, it means you are destroying your country.

— Malala Yousafzai

Unfortunately, due to lack of public funding, research on WFPB nutrition intervention for cancer is scarce to non-existent. And as Dr. Campbell stated, "It's only going to get worse because industry is taking over independent government-funded studies. No pharmaceutical company is going to fund studies like this unless they can patent it and put it in a pill."

Currently, the only study independently funded (by the NIH), investigating the use of WFPB nutrition to treat recurrent cancer I am aware of is being conducted by Dr. T. Colin Campbell's son, Dr. Thomas Campbell, MD, at the University of Rochester, NY. Here is the summary of the study, cut and pasted from PubMed:

> This research will examine the feasibility of conducting a strict whole-food, plant-based dietary intervention in women with stable metastatic breast cancer currently undergoing conventional treatments. In addition, this research will provide preliminary data on dietary intakes and the effect of plant-based nutrition on numerous outcomes reflecting cancer prognosis and overall health using advanced imaging, various blood biomarkers linked to cancer progression, and numerous symptom questionnaires.

Sounds like a great study to me, and I look forward to seeing the results! It's a randomized controlled trial of recurrent breast cancer patients using plant-based nutrition. It's a small study (60 people total) and fairly short in duration (six weeks of intervention), but should be comprehensive and long enough to determine if it moves the needle on recurrent breast cancer. The study is underway as of this writing and is scheduled to be completed in December of 2020. As a side note, Thomas Campbell has also written an excellent book on transitioning to a plant- based diet entitled *The Campbell Plan*. Buy it and read it!

The AICR is in the process of funding additional research on treating cancer with diet, and you can find the details on their website (https://www.aicr.org/research/projects/).

Chapter 37 – Going Forward

When I first found out I had prostate cancer in 2011, my doctor told me that many treatments and possibly a cure were in the pipeline. Maybe in five years, my recurrent prostate cancer would be curable. Well, I am nine years in, and I am not holding my breath for a "cure." What I want is long term suppression. I am doing everything within my control to create an environment in my body where the cancer is not happy. I most likely will always have cancer, but that doesn't mean that cancer will defeat me.

Summary

1. Although there is limited research on WFPB eating and PC, what we do know is profound.
2. We don't need policy to catch up with research to take action now. The best available scientific evidence to date demonstrates the healthiest way to eat is a WFPB diet without added salt, sugar, or oil.
3. Step out of that comfort box—it may be what got you here in the first place.

CHAPTER 38
WHAT I DO EVERY DAY

This isn't just "another day, another dollar." It's more like "another day, another miracle.

— Victoria Moran

Here's what I do in general on a daily basis after almost nine years post-diagnosis:

I get enough sleep! Usually, nine hours a night when not traveling or working. I never slept as well as I do now, and I give a lot of credit to cannabis.

I usually wake up around 8:00 a.m. Mindy brings me breakfast in bed, so I'll stay there and get some writing done. I will work in bed sometimes until 10:30 or 11:00 a.m. I get a lot done in there, OK?

I always drink two full glasses of water when I wake up before anything else. Then I have my morning "elixir" of modified citrus pectin, apple peel powder, freshly ground black cumin, dandelion root, matcha, milk thistle, and mushroom powder. All these ingredients have been shown to have anti-cancer properties. This drink is anything but "delicious," but I have learned to like it, grit and all. THEN, I have my first cup of coffee with a tiny bit of organic soy milk. I usually drink two to three cups before noon. I also usually have a cup or two of green tea in the afternoon. No more caffeine after that.

Breakfast is very simple and almost always the same:

> A bowl of hot boiled intact grains (soaked overnight and then boiled) of oat, farro, kamut, buckwheat, or sorghum with a little unsweetened soy milk topped with fresh or frozen organic berries (think Costco for both!), topped with two tablespoons of freshly ground (coffee grinder) flax seeds for my Omega-3's. I put a little maple syrup on to sweeten it up. Maple syrup is basically sugar with little or no nutrients, but it IS delicious!

Mid-morning snack: Usually nothing but occasionally one of Mindy's black bean brownies (OMG!) or a few of her signature garbanzo bean cookies (made from whole garbanzo beans—the recipe is in her book, *The Plant Powered Penis)*.

Lunch usually is between 12:30 and 1:30 p.m. and consists of a big salad (usually from a wholefoods salad bar if we are traveling) and a legume soup (split pea or lentil). For lunch, all I drink is water.

Chapter 38 – What I Do Every Day

Mid-afternoon snack: For some reason, I get a hankering for citrus around 2:00 p.m., so I eat a whole orange or tangerine.

I usually wrap up my work (or surf) day around 4:00 p.m. but usually return to research around 7:00 p.m. Also, around 4:00 p.m., I take a very precise oral dose of cannabis oil which is a 1:1 ratio of THC:CBD, just like Dr. Donald Abrams recommends to his cancer patients. The THC buzz will not kick in for another hour or so, and this is when I usually do 20 to 30 minutes of sitting meditation with light background music (I LOVE this part of the day because I ALWAYS feel better after meditating). After meditation (if there is no surf or I am not in a SURF zone, both of which is most of the time), I'll work out for around 45 minutes to an hour. My work out is usually a jog of two to three miles followed by some upper body strength training and squats. Upper body strength training is in a gym if I am at a hotel. If I don't have equipment, (and I usually don't), it's pushups and tricep dips on a bench. Chin ups if I have access to a chin-up bar.

By this time, usually around 5:30 p.m., my cannabis buzz begins to make an appearance. This is CRITICAL! As I mentioned earlier in the book, I had a lifelong habit of making and drinking at least two martinis every day, and the Pavlovian martini bell STILL starts to ring around five p.m. in my brain. But when the THC begins to have an impact, I don't NEED a martini. (I never needed one, just always wanted one and had one or two). Instead, I make myself a hibiscus tea and sip it while I make dinner and listen to music. I am usually the one making dinner because I love to cook. Mindy, not so much, which is just fine because she is usually working on our work schedule while I cook. We have several variations on the same dinner theme, but it is always simple. The best way I can describe our dinner fare is…… rice (or congee) with lentils or some kind of beans, either a roasted purple or orange sweet potato, a small salad, and organic corn tortillas grilled in the oven WITHOUT OIL. That's it. Sometimes we will make a stir fry, whole grain pasta with red sauce, sometimes just a salad. Check out our website (https://onedaytowellness.org/recipe-categories/) for tons of easy to prepare WFPB no oil recipes!

I usually just drink water for dinner along with some herbal tea, but sometimes I will have a glass of red wine with Mindy as a special treat which is a few times a week.

After the dishes are done, it's usually 6:30 or 7:00 p.m., and I'm feeling relaxed and……. well……. I get the munchies! To satisfy my cannabis-induced desire to eat more, I will almost always have a few pieces of toast (made from fresh-baked whole grain bread—the recipe is on our website) (https://onedaytowellness.org/recipe-categories/) with fresh homemade LOW-FAT roasted chestnut butter (also on the site) topped with mango, papaya, or berries. We made the transition from almond to chestnut butter

Chapter 38 – What I Do Every Day

because chestnuts are only 10% fat compared to 75% in almonds, and the taste is every bit as delicious.

I TRY to STOP eating by 7:00 p.m. based on the guidance of Dr. Greger and Dr. Klaper, but this can be a struggle! Sometimes dessert doesn't get eaten until 7:30. Regardless, it's the last thing I eat before I go to bed, and I do not snack or eat anything after dessert is done.

When we are at home in Santa Cruz, Mindy and I go for a walk/run after dinner every night, weather permitting. We run a little, walk a little, maybe do some leg lifts and pushups on a bench. It's usually less than an hour, but the light physical activity post-dinner is an excellent way to set yourself up for a great night's sleep.

Sometimes we will watch a documentary or a TV show before bed, but not nearly as often as we used to. I get into bed around 9:00 p.m., read some of a trashy novel, watch some surf porn (It's a nice respite from doing cancer research all day!) and kill the lights by 10:00 p.m.

That is a typical activity/meal day for us. We never count calories, macronutrients, or any other dieting trick. I eat all I want, more or less when I want. I never gain or lose weight (except during fasting), and I LOVE the food. I'll never go back to my old eating habits. I have lost all of my desire for crap food, and I crave healthy food because it makes me feel awesome. Period!

Every change I have made outlined in this book since my diagnosis has had a direct, measurable positive outcome for me. None have turned out to be a negative. Additionally, in the beginning, all these lifestyle changes and behavioral tweaks I have discussed in the preceding pages seemed... overwhelming. And in each case, I discovered my fear of change was unfounded. That FEAR was the ONLY thing between me and a better life and a better ME. Push the fear of change aside, ask yourself, "What have I got to lose and what do I have to gain," and then dive in. Big changes, big results, across the board. Let me know how you do!

Don't wait until science catches up with your disease. Regular exercise, stress reduction, and a low-fat, high-fiber, plant-based diet are good for anyone's general health, and they make an obvious addition to any prostate cancer treatment program.

EPILOGUE

I choose to be happy.

— Bruce Mylrea

"All roads for you lead to Lupron," my local oncologist told me recently. Probably, but I am in no hurry. I'll most likely be back on hormone therapy in the near future, but I will mull it over before proceeding. I'm doing everything I can possibly do myself to slow down my cancer progression. I know I'm not doing it all right, but I am determined to give it my best effort, and so far, it feels great.

Let's see what the PSMA scan says..... BUT WAIT, FIRST THIS IMPORTANT ANNOUNCEMENT:

> The world is a different place than it was when I wrote the previous chapter. The PSMA scan has been cancelled indefinitely, along with every other activity on the planet. COVID 19 is shaking modern humanity to its core as I write this. It cannot be put into words. UCLA has no idea

when they can reschedule my PSMA scan that I have now waited three months for.

It's Monday, March 16th. Thich Nhat Hanh says that all we have is the present moment, but for the last eight and a half years, it has been a constant struggle for me to remember that. I look internally, I FEEL internally, in the present moment, right now, in perfect physical shape. In the present moment, there is nothing wrong with me. Everything is right. But once again, I am pulled from the present to contemplate a rising PSA without knowing when I can actually peer inside again. Maybe it doesn't matter. In light of Corona, my situation seems almost trivial. But the circumstances are still crushing for me personally.

But I am happy. I confront mortality every day, and it has made me much more alive, emotional, sensitive, and caring. I have learned that the only true path to happiness is helping others with their suffering. I hope I am helping YOU! The shocking wake-up call of PC is a reminder that our existence on this planet is short and getting shorter every day. I have awakened, and if it took a life-threatening PC diagnosis, so be it. A great life and happiness are available to all of us, but we have to acknowledge and take responsibility for the behaviors we need to change in order to achieve it. I promise it's there for you, me, and anyone in any condition. Choose to be happy!

THE END (or the beginning, I hope!)

Summary

1. Cancer sucks, but how you deal with it is entirely up to you.
2. You have more power than you might think you do.
3. Don't leave any cards on the table. Make the right choice now to live your best life.

GLOSSARY OF TERMS AND ACRONYMS

ACE – American Council on Exercise.

ACLM – American College of Lifestyle Medicine.

ADT – Androgen Deprivation Therapy.

AFPA – American Federation of Professional Athletes.

AICR – American Institute for Cancer Research.

ALA - Alpha-Linolenic Acid.

Allopathic – Relating to or being a system of medicine that aims to combat disease by using remedies (such as drugs or surgery) that produce effects that are different from or incompatible with those of the disease being treated.

Allopathic care – The treatment involved with the suppression of symptoms which are manifestations of certain pathologies.

ADA – American Dietetic Association.

AMA – American Medical Association.

AND – Academy of Nutrition and Dietetics.

APC – Advanced Prostate Cancer.

Apoptosis – The death of cells which occurs as a normal and controlled part of an organism's growth or development. It is cell death via shrinkage. Cancer cells are just the opposite—they don't have cell death, they have uncontrollable growth and produce a protein that blocks apoptosis. It was found that cannabis kills tumor cells and increases apoptosis.

ASCO – American Society of Clinical Oncology.

Autophagy – A mechanism in cancerous cells that improves the resistance of cancer cells to radiation. Once these autophagy-related genes are inhibited, cancer cell death is potentiated.

BPH – Benign Prostatic Hyperplasia – An enlarged prostate.

Big Pharma – The nickname given to the world's pharmaceutical industry. It also includes the trade group, Pharmaceutical Research and Manufacturers of America (PhRMA).

Biopsy – An examination of tissue removed from a living body to discover the presence, cause, or extent of a disease.

BMC – Block Medical Center of Integrative Oncology (in Chicago)

BMI – Body Mass Index - The BMI is a measure of body fat based on height and weight that applies to adult men and women. It provides a reliable indicator of body fatness and is used to screen for weight categories that may lead to health problems.

BMJ – *British Medical Journal.*

BPH – Benign Prostatic Hyperplasia (hypertrophy) – An enlargement of the prostate gland.

Brachytherapy Techniques – A type of internal radiation therapy for treating cancer. Seeds, ribbons, or capsules that contain a radiation source are placed the patient's body, in or near the cancer. It is a local treatment and treats only a specific part of your body.

Bump – refers to a problem of any type such as a conflict, decision, dilemma, disagreement, disappointment, frustration, issue, upsetting interaction, or stress.

Bump Theory – embraces the idea that internal thoughts exert strong influence on how challenging life situations are handled.

Cannabis – Also known as marijuana. A tall plant with a stiff upright stem, divided serrated leaves, and glandular hairs. It is sometimes used as a drug to ease pain and inflammation and help control spasms and seizures. It was found that cannabis kills tumor cells and increases aptosis.

CaPSURE™ – UCSF Cancer of the Prostate Strategic Urologic Research Endeavor—a longitudinal, observational study of approximately 15,000 men with all stages of biopsy-proven prostate cancer. Patients have enrolled at 43 community urology practices, academic medical centers, and VA hospitals throughout the United States since 1995.

Case Control Study – Observational study in which two existing groups differing in outcome are identified and compared on the basis of some supposed causal attribute.

CAT Scan – Computerized Axial Tomography Scan – an X-ray image made using a form of tomography in which a computer controls the motion of the X-ray source and detectors, processes the data, and produces the image. CAT scans are a crucial part of the cancer diagnosis and cancer treatment process; it takes X-ray images from multiple angles. This allows doctors to see where the cancer is located and determine whether the cancer treatment is working. They are less detailed than MRI scans.

CBD – Short for cannabidiol, a chemical compound from the cannabis Sativa plant, which is also known as marijuana or help, according to the US National Library of Medicine. CBD may help reduce symptoms related to cancer and side effects related to cancer treatment.

CDC – Centers for Disease Control.

Cellular Oxidation – A process that takes place which is fundamental to the life of cells that require energy and oxygen. Oils slow the process and impair artery function.

Cohort Study (1) – A longitudinal study that samples a cohort (a group of people who share a defining characteristic, typically those who experienced a common event in a selected period, such as prostate cancer), and performs a cross-section at intervals through time.

Cohort Study (2) – A longitudinal study used in medicine which is an analysis of risk factors. It follows a group of people who do not have the disease and uses correlations to determine the risk of subject contraction.

Congee – Boiled, intact whole grains.

COSA – Clinical Oncology Society of Australia.

Cross Sectional Study - An observational study that analyzes data from a population, or a representative subset, at a specific point in time.

CRP – C-Reactive Protein, a substance produced by the liver in response to inflammation. CRP levels also have been linked to cancer and its aggressiveness.

CVD – Cardiovascular Disease.

Cytotoxic – Of, relating to, or producing a toxic effect on cells, cell-killing. An agent or process that kills cells such as chemotherapy and radiotherapy which are forms of cytotoxic therapy. Fasting manipulates pathways and can make cancer cells more susceptible to standard cytotoxic treatment with radiation and chemotherapy.

DHA – Docosahexaenoic Acid – An Omega-3 fatty acid that has many important functions, including making up a significant portion of brain tissue, cerebral cortex, skin, and retina. Higher intake of Omega-3 fats such as DHA has been linked to lower risk of several cancers, including colorectal, pancreatic, breast, and prostate cancer. DHA may help reduce cancer risk through its anti-inflammatory effects. (See "EPA" below.)

EBRT – External Beam Radiation Therapy.

EBERT – External Beam Electron Radiation Therapy.

ECA – East Coast Alliance for Aerobic & Fitness Professionals.

ED – Erectile Dysfunction

EFA – Essential Fatty Acid.

EPA – Eicosapentaenoic Acid–used in combination with DHA (see DHA above) in fish oil preparations for a variety of conditions, including prostate cancer, to help maintain body weight in people with cancer, and to reduce the side effect of chemotherapy in people with cancer.

EPIC – European Prospective Investigation into Cancer and Nutrition Study.

Epidemiology – The branch of medical science dealing with the incidence, distribution, transmission, and control of disease.

FAO – Food and Agriculture Organization of the United Nations.

Finasteride – A medication used by the medical profession to shrink an enlarged prostate (benign prostatic hyperplasia or BPH) in adult men. It may be

Glossary of Terms and Acronyms

used alone or taken in combination with other medications to reduce symptoms of BPH

Flexitarians – People who eat meat more on a weekly basis rather than daily.

Ga PET (Ga PET Scan – A PET scan (see PET and PET scan below) with Gallium (a radiopharmaceutical tracer) used during PET scans for evaluating primary and metastatic cancer.

GBD – Global Burden of Disease Study.

GBM – Glioblastoma Multiforme is aggressive cancer of the brain.

Glioblastoma Multiforme (GBM) – is the most aggressive type of cancer that begins within the brain.

HCA – Hydroxycarboxylic Acid – A cancer-causing metabolite found in cooked beef and a by-product of grilling any animal meat at high temperatures.

HIV – Human Immunodeficiency Virus.

Homeostasis – The ability or tendency of the body or a cell to seek and maintain a condition of equilibrium—a stable internal environment—as it deals with external changes. The ability to maintain a steady body temperature is an example of homeostasis.

HT – Hormone Therapy.

IACR – International Agency for Cancer Research.

IGF-1 – Insulin-like growth hormone-1.

IMTG – Intramyocellular Triacylglycerol.

Integrative Medicine – a form of medical therapy that combines practices and treatments from alternative medicine with conventional medicine

Integrative Nutrition® – a concept trademarked by the Institute for Integrative Nutrition® that states that food is not just about physical nutrition, but also has an emotional, mental, and spiritual component.

Integrative Oncology – is a patient-centered, evidence-informed field of cancer care that utilizes mind and body practices, natural products, and/or lifestyle modifications from different traditions alongside conventional cancer treatments. Integrative oncology aims to optimize health, quality of life, and clinical outcomes across the cancer care continuum and to empower people to prevent cancer and become active participants before, during, and beyond cancer treatment.

Intramyocellular fat – Also known as intramuscular triglycerides, intramuscular triacylglycerol, or intramyocellular triacylglycerol (IMTG), is located inside skeletal muscle fibers. It is stored in lipid droplets that exist in close proximity to the mitochondria, where it serves as an energy store that can be used during exercise.

Isoflavones – A group of phytochemicals discovered to inhibit the growth of prostate cancer in mice.

JAMA – *Journal of the American Medical Association* – A medical journal published 48 times a year by the American Medical Association. It publishes original research, reviews, and editorials covering all aspects of biomedicine.

Ketone – A chemical substance that the body makes when it does not have enough insulin in the blood. When ketones build up in the body for a long time, serious illness or coma can result.

Ketosis – A metabolic state characterized by raised levels of ketone bodies in the body tissues, which is typically pathological in conditions such as diabetes, or may be the consequence of a diet that is very low in carbohydrates.

LA – Linoleic Acid.

LACE – Life After Cancer Epidemiology (LACE) Study. A cohort of early breast cancer survivors (United States).

LNCaP Cells – Lymph-Node Carcinoma (Cancer) of the Prostate – LNCaP cells are a cell line of human cells commonly used in the field of oncology. They are androgen-sensitive human prostate adenocarcinoma cells, have weakly-adherent qualities, and grow well in vitro, albeit slowly, and can be grown in aggregates or as individual cells.

Long-Term Statin Regime – Protects against prostate cancer death.

Longitudinal Study – A research design that involves repeated observations of the same variables (e.g., people) over short or long periods of time.

Marijuana – Also known as cannabis –Sometimes used as a drug to ease pain and inflammation and help control spasms and seizures. It was found that marijuana kills tumor cells and increases aptosis.

Meta-analysis – Combines the results of multiple scientific studies.

MRI – Magnetic Resonance Imaging – a medical imaging technique used in radiology to form pictures of the anatomy and the physiological processes of the body. They are more detailed than CAT scans.

Nadar – Lowest point.

NCI – National Cancer Institute.

ng/mL – Nanograms per milliliter, a measurement often used for lab test results. Research shows that an increase of .75 ng/mL a year is an early indicator of prostate cancer if a man has a total PSA result between 4.0 and 10.0 ng/mL. Further, an increase of 2.0 ng/mL over a year period predicts a higher likelihood of death due to aggressive prostate cancer.

NHS – National Health Service.

NIH – National Institute of Health.

ODTW – One Day to Wellness (onedaytowellness.org)— Bruce and Mindy's site covering evidence-based nutrition, offering simple, easy-to-implement evidence-based behavioral change tools.

Omnivore – A person who eats both animal and vegetable substances.

Oncologist – A medical practitioner (specialist) who practices oncology; someone qualified to diagnose and treat cancer.

Oncology – A branch of medicine that deals with the prevention, diagnosis, and treatment of cancer.

PAC (1) – Polycyclic Aromatic Hydrocarbons are components in tobacco smoke and outdoor and indoor air pollution that have a great negative impact on humans and the environment, and can cause cancer in humans.

PAC (2) – Polycyclic Aromatic Hydrocarbon – A cancer-causing metabolite found in cooked beef and a by-product of grilling any animal meat at high temperatures.

PC – Prostate Cancer—the development of cancer in the prostate, a gland in the male reproductive system.

PCF – Prostate Cancer Foundation.

PCRI – Prostate Cancer Research Institute.

Pescatarian – See Pesco-Vegetarian below.

Pesco-Vegetarian – A vegetarian who also consumes fish and seafood, making his/her diet a type of semi-vegetarian diet. Adding seafood to an otherwise vegetarian diet can make it easier to meet one's nutrient needs while still maintaining a mainly plant-based diet.

PET – Positive Emission Tomography (x-rays or ultrasound).

PET/CT – Positron Emission Tomography/Computed Tomography.

PET Scan – A specialized radiology procedure (imaging test) that helps reveal how body tissues and organs are functioning. It uses a radioactive drug (tracer) to show this activity to detect, examine, identify, and/or follow the progress of certain conditions such as cancer. It is a type of nuclear medicine procedure.

PhRMA – Pharmaceutical Research and Manufacturers of America, part of the Big Pharma group. (See Big Pharma above.)

Phytochemicals (chemicals only found in plant food) – Plant-based chemicals which have many disease-fighting compounds that strengthen our immune system, repel viral attacks in our bodies, and mitigate cancer initiation and progression.

PMSA Scan – Prostate Specific Membrane Antigen Scan – A scan used either in the diagnosis or follow-up of prostate cancer. It can show cancer activity in the prostate, surrounding tissue, lymph glands, or bone and can help assess cancer spread and response to therapy.

PPC – PlantPure Communities.

PROS – Prostate Oncology Specialists.

PSA – Prostate Specific Antigen—an antigenic enzyme released by the prostate and found in abnormally high concentrations in the blood of men with prostate cancer.

PSMA - Prostate Specific Membrane Antigen, a useful diagnostic and possibly therapeutic target for prostate cancer.

PUFA – PolyUnsaturated Fatty Acid.

RCT – Randomized Controlled Trial.

REDUCE Study – A Clinical Research Study To Reduce The Incidence Of Prostate Cancer In Men Who Are At Increased Risk.

Research Study – A systematic approach that a researcher uses to conduct a scientific study. It is the overall synchronization of identified components and data resulting in a plausible outcome.

ROS – Reactive Oxygen Species – sometimes referred to as "A Dance with the Devil." They have a dual role in cancer… they can promote facilitating cancer cell proliferation, and on the other hand can promote stress-induced cancer cell death.

RP – Radical Prostatectomy—A surgical procedure that removes the prostate gland and attached seminal vesicles.

RSO – Rick Simpson Oil – a cannabis oil made from the marijuana plant containing high amounts of THC (tetrahydrocannabinol), the active compound in marijuana.

SAD – Standard American Diet.

SELECT - The 2012 Selenium and Vitamin E Cancer Prevention Trial, the largest prostate cancer prevention study to date.

SOS free – Salt, Oil, and Sugar free.

STF – Short Term Fasting

Study – See Cohort study (1), Cohort study (2), Longitudinal Study, Research Study.

Temozolomide – Chemotherapy.

THC – Short for tetrahydrocannabinol, a chemical compound found in the cannabis (marijuana) plant.

TIP – A combination of chemotherapy drugs (paclitaxel, ifosfamide, and cisplatin) originally developed as a first-line salvage chemotherapy for testicular cancer that has spread or come back.

TMAO – Trimethylamine N-oxide promotes the formation of cholesterol plaques in our blood vessels, and is directly implicated in the progression of atherosclerosis and other chronic diseases. It may be linked to death from prostate cancer.

TNHC – TrueNorth Health Center.

Tomography – a technique for displaying a representation of a cross section through a human body or other solid object using X-rays or ultrasound.

UCLA – The University of California, Los Angeles.

UCSD – The University of California, San Diego.

Glossary of Terms and Acronyms

UCSF – University of California at San Francisco.

UCSF Cancer of the Prostate Strategic Urologic Research Endeavor – See CaPSURE™.

USC – University of Southern California.

USDA – United States Dept. of Agriculture.

USPSTF – U.S. Preventive Services Task Force.

VEGF – Vascular Endothelial Growth Factor—a potential target for the treatment of cancer. It is an important protein that helps to create blood and lymph vessels. This unique protein can help tumors thrive, and when used correctly, may also work in cancer treatments.

WCRF – World Cancer Research Fund.

WF – Whole Foods—food that has been processed or refined as little as possible and is free from additives or other artificial substances.

WFPB – Whole Foods, Plant-Based—A way of eating that focuses on nutrient dense, whole plant foods. The term "whole" in WFPB describes foods that are minimally processed.

WFPB SOS-free – Whole Foods, Plant-Based, with no ADDED salt, oil, sugar.

WFPBD – Whole Foods, Plant-Based Diet—a diet consisting mostly or entirely of foods derived from plants, including vegetables, grains, nuts, seeds, legumes, and fruits and with few or no animal products.

WHO – World Health Organization.

WOF – Water-only fasting.

EDUCATIONAL AND RECIPE RESOURCES

American Institute of Cancer Research: https://www.aicr.org/

Barnard, Dr. Neil. Physicians Committee for Responsible Medicine: https://www.pcrm.org/

Block Center for Integrated Oncology: http://blockmd.com/

Campbell, Dr. T. Colin: NutritionStudies.org. https://nutritionstudies.org/about/dr-t-colin-campbell/

Chef AJ: https://www.chefajwebsite.com/index.html

Cochrane Collaboration: https://www.chefajwebsite.com/index.html

Food Revolution Network: http://foodrevolution.org/

Fred Hutchinson Cancer Research Center: fredhutch.org

Greger, Dr. Michael. Nutrition Facts.org: https://nutritionfacts.org/

McDougall, Dr. John: https://www.drmcdougall.com

Mylrea, Bruce and Mindy. One Day to Wellness: https://onedaytowellness.org/

PlantPure Nation: https://www.plantpurenation.com/pages/about-the-film

Prostate Cancer Foundation: https://www.pcf.org/

Prostate Cancer Research Institute: https://pcri.org/

Pubmed Online. NIH National Library of Medicine: https://pubmed.ncbi.nlm.nih.gov/

UC San Diego School of Medicine, Center For Integrated Medicine: https://medschool.ucsd.edu/som/fmph/research/cim/pages/default.aspx

UCSF Osher Center for Integrative Medicine, Integrative Cancer Care https://osher.ucsf.edu/patient-care/treatments/integrative-cancer-care

World Cancer Research Fund International: https://www.wcrf.org/

World Health Organization: https://www.who.int/

REFERENCES

PART ONE

Chapter 2

1. PubMed, NIH, National Library of Medicine. "Global, Regional, and National Cancer Incidence, Mortality, Years of Life Lost, Years Lived with Disability, and Disability-Adjusted Life-years for 32 Cancer Groups, 1990 to 2015: A Systematic Analysis for the Global Burden of Disease Study." Global Burden of Disease Cancer Collaboration; Christina Fitzmaurice, Tomi F. Akinyemiju, Faris Hasan Al Lami, et al. 2018.
https://pubmed.ncbi.nlm.nih.gov/29860482/
2. Journal of Biomedical Education. "The State of Nutrition Education at US Medical Schools." Kelly M. Adams, W. Scott Butsch, Martin Kohlmeier. August 2015.
https://www.hindawi.com/journals/jbe/2015/357627/
3. American Medical Association. "What's at stake in nutrition education during med school." July 2015.

https://www.ama-assn.org/education/accelerating-change-medical-education/whats-stake-nutrition-education-during-med-school
4. *Journal of the National Cancer Institute.* "Hans Christian Andersen and the Value of New Cancer Treatments." Richard L. Schilsky, Lowell E. Schnipper. December 13, 2017. https://academic.oup.com/jnci/article/110/5/441/4735107

Chapter 4

1. World Cancer Research Fund, American Institute for Cancer Research. "Global cancer data by country: Exploring which countries have the highest cancer rates." F. Bray, J. Ferlay, I. Soerjomataram, et al. 2018. https://www.wcrf.org/dietandcancer/cancer-trends/data-cancer-frequency-country
2. Research Gate. "Emerging proteomics biomarkers and prostate cancer burden in Africa." Figure 1: Global epidemiology of prostate cancer showing high burden of prostate cancer in Africa." September 2018. https://www.researchgate.net/figure/Global-epidemiology-of-prostate-cancer-showing-high-burden-of-prostate-cancer-in-Africa_fig1_314117229

References - Part One

3. PMC, US National Library of Medicine, National Institutes of Health. "A Western Dietary Pattern Increases Prostate Cancer Risk: A Systematic Review and meta-Analysis." Robert Fabiani, Liliana Minelli, Gaia Bertarelli, Silvia Bacci. Oct. 2016.
https://www.ncbi.nlm.nih.gov/pmc/articles/PMC5084014/

4. World Cancer Research Fund, American Institute for Cancer Research. "Prostate cancer statistics: Prostate cancer is the second most common cancer in men worldwide." F. Bray, J. Ferlay, I. Soerjomataram, et al. 2018.
https://www.wcrf.org/dietandcancer/cancer-trends/prostate-cancer-statistics

Chapter 10

1. *Harvard Health Publishing,* Harvard Medical School. "Exercise as a part of cancer treatment." Monique Tello, MD MPH.
https://www.health.harvard.edu/blog/exercise-as-part-of-cancer-treatment-2018061314035

Chapter 14

1. PubMed, NIH, National Library of Medicine. "Feasibility, Acceptability and Preliminary Psychological Benefits of Mindfulness Meditation Training in a Sample of Men Diagnosed with Prostate Cancer on Active Surveillance:

Results from a Randomized Controlled Pilot Trial." August 2017.
https://pubmed.ncbi.nlm.nih.gov/27145355/

Chapter 15

1. The Lancet Regional Health. "Alcohol use and burden for 195 countries and territories, 1990–2016: a systematic analysis for the Global Burden of Disease Study 2016. "M. Ezzati, S. V. Hoorn, A. D. Lopez, et al. August, 2018.
https://www.thelancet.com/article/S0140-6736(18)31310-2/fulltext

Chapter 19

1. *Journal of the American College of Cardiology.* "Consumption of Saturated Fat Impairs the Anti-Inflammatory Properties of High-Density Lipproteins and Endothelial Function." Stephen J. Nicholls, Pia Lundman, Jason A. Harmer, et al. August 2006.
https://www.sciencedirect.com/science/article/pii/S0735109706013386
2. Elsevier: *The American Journal of Cardiology.* "Effect of a Single High-Fat Meal on Endothelial Function in Healthy Subjects." Robert A. Vogel, Mary C. Corretti, Gary D. Plotnick. February 1997.
 https://www.thelancet.com/article/S0140-6736(18)31310-2/fulltext

Chapter 25

1. TrueNorth Health Center. "British Medical Journal publishes Report from TNH on the Successful Treatment of Lymphoma Cancer with Fasting and a Vegan, SOS-free Diet." Alan Goldhamer DC, Michael Klaper MD, Afsoon Foorohar DO, Toshia R. Myers Ph.D. December 2015.
https://www.healthpromoting.com/learning-center/articles/british-medical-journal-publishes-report-tnh-successful-treatment-lymphoma

PART TWO

Chapter 28

1. American Cancer Society. "Diet and Physical Activity: What's the Cancer Connection?" June 2014 (Revised April 2017).
https://www.cancer.org/cancer/cancer-causes/diet-physical-activity/diet-and-physical-activity.html

Chapter 29

1. National Geographic 2nd edition (sold by Amazon.com). *The Blue Zones, Second Edition: 9 Lessons for Living Longer from the*

People Who've Lived the Longest. Dan Buettner. November 2012.
https://www.amazon.com/Blue-Zones-Second-Lessons-Longest/dp/1426209487/ref=tmm_pap_swatch_0?_encoding=UTF8&qid=&sr=

2. PubMed, NIH, National Library of Medicine. "Risk Factors for Prostate Carcinoma in Taiwan: A Case-Control Study in a Chinese Population." J. F. Sung, R. S. Lin, Y. S. Pu, et al. August 1999.
https://pubmed.ncbi.nlm.nih.gov/10430257/

3. PubMed, NIH, National Library of Medicine. "Case-control Study of Diet and Prostate Cancer in China." M. M. Lee, R. T. Wang, A, W. Hsing, et al. Dec. 1998.
https://pubmed.ncbi.nlm.nih.gov/10189039/

4. PubMed, NIH, National Library of Medicine. "Re: Trends in Mortality from Cancers of the Breast, Colon, Prostate, Esophagus, and Stomach in East Asia: Role of Nutrition Transition." Patrick C. Walsh. 2012.
https://pubmed.ncbi.nlm.nih.gov/22682827/

5. PubMed, NIH, National Library of Medicine. "The Experience of Japan as a Clue to the Etiology of Testicular and Prostatic Cancers." D. Ganmaa, X. M. Li, L. Q. Qin, P. Y. Wang, et al.
https://pubmed.ncbi.nlm.nih.gov/12710911/

Chapter 30

1. American Institute for Cancer Research. "Cancer Resource: Living with Cancer." https://store.aicr.org/collections/cancer-survivors/products/cancer-resource-living-with-cancer
2. PubMed, NIH, National Library of Medicine. "REDUCE" - A Clinical Research Study to Reduce the Incidence of Prostate Cancer in Men Who Are at Increased Risk. Glaxo Smith Kline. March 2020 (Updated September 2016). https://clinicaltrials.gov/ct2/show/NCT00056407
3. *Science Daily.* "Obesity Is Risk Factor for Aggressive Prostate Cancer." Medical College of Georgia. May 2005. https://www.sciencedaily.com/releases/2005/05/050523091709.htm
4. Nature Research, Nature Reviews Cancer. "Cytokines in cancer pathogenesis and cancer therapy." Glenn Dranoff 2004. https://www.nature.com/articles/nrc1252
5. PMC, US National Library of Medicine, National Institutes of Health. "Vegetarian diets and incidence of diabetes in the Adventist health Study-2." S. Tonstad, K. Stewart, K. Oda, et al. October 2011. https://www.ncbi.nlm.nih.gov/pmc/articles/PMC3638849/

6. PubMed, NIH, National Library of Medicine. "The BROAD Study: A Randomised Controlled Trial Using a Whole Food Plant-Based Diet in the Community for Obesity, Ischaemic Heart Disease or Diabetes." N. Wright, L. Wilson, M. Smith, et al. March 2017.
https://pubmed.ncbi.nlm.nih.gov/28319109/

Chapter 31

1. PMC, US National Library of Medicine, National Institutes of Health. "We Can Prevent and Even Reverse Coronary Artery Heart Disease." Caldwell B. Esselstyn, Jr. August 2007.
https://www.ncbi.nlm.nih.gov/pmc/articles/PMC2100124/
2. Physicians Committee for Responsible Medicine. "A plant-based diet is a powerful tool for **preventing, managing,** and even **reversing** type 2 diabetes." Neal Barnard.
https://www.pcrm.org/health-topics/diabetes/
3. PubMed, NIH, National Library of Medicine. "Intensive Lifestyle Changes for Reversal of Coronary Heart Disease." D. Ornish, L. W. Scherwitz, J. H. Billings, et al. December 1998.
https://pubmed.ncbi.nlm.nih.gov/9863851/
4. PubMed, NIH, National Library of Medicine. "Resolving the Coronary Artery Disease Epidemic Through Plant-Based Nutrition." C. B.

Esselstyn Jr. Autumn 2001.
https://pubmed.ncbi.nlm.nih.gov/11832674/
5. PubMed, NIH, National Library of Medicine. "A Plant-Based Diet in Overweight Individual in a 16-week Randomized Clinical Trial: Metabolic Benefits of Plant Protein." Hana Kahleova, Rebecca Fleeman, Adela Hlozkova, et al. November 2018.
https://pubmed.ncbi.nlm.nih.gov/30405108/
6. The Journal of Urology. "Intensive Lifestyle Changes May Affect the Progression of Prostate Cancer." Dean Ornish, Gerdi Weidner, William R. Fair, et al. September 2005.
https://www.sciencedirect.com/science/article/abs/pii/S0022534701685185.
7. Centers for Disease Control and Prevention. National Center for Health Statistics. "Dietary intake for adults aged 20 and over." 2018. https://www.cdc.gov/nchs/fastats/diet.htm
8. PubMed, NIH, National Library of Medicine. "Intensive Lifestyle Changes May Affect the Progression of Prostate Cancer." Dean Ornish, Gerdi Weidner, William R. Fair, et al. September 2005.
https://www.sciencedirect.com/science/article/abs/pii/S0022534701685185
9. PubMed, NIH, National Library of Medicine. "A Dietary Intervention for Recurrent Prostate Cancer After Definitive Primary Treatment:

Results of a Randomized Pilot Trial." James Carmody, Barbara Olendzki, George Reed, et al. December 2008.
https://pubmed.ncbi.nlm.nih.gov/18400281/

10. PMC, US National Library of Medicine, National Institutes of Health. "Biological Mediators of Effect of Diet and Stress Reduction on Prostate Cancer." Gordon A. Saxe, Jacqueline M. Major, Lindsey Westerberg, et al. August 2009.
https://www.ncbi.nlm.nih.gov/pmc/articles/PMC2733349/

11. PubMed, NIH, National Library of Medicine, Clinical Trials.gov. "Diet in Altering Disease Progression in Patients with Prostate Cancer on Active Surveillance." November 2010 (Updated March 2019).
https://clinicaltrials.gov/ct2/show/NCT01238172

Chapter 32

1. PubMed, NIH, National Library of Medicine. "Risk Factors for Prostate Carcinoma in Taiwan: A Case-Control Study in a Chinese Population." J. F. Sung, R. S. Lin, Y. S. Pu, et al. August 1999.
https://pubmed.ncbi.nlm.nih.gov/10430257/

2. PubMed, NIH, National Library of Medicine. "Case-control Study of Diet and Prostate

Cancer in China." M. M. Lee, R. T. Wang, A. W. Hsing, et al. December 1998.
https://pubmed.ncbi.nlm.nih.gov/10189039/
3. PubMed, NIH, National Library of Medicine. "Trends in Mortality from Cancers of the Breast, Colon, Prostate, Esophagus, and Stomach in East Asia: Role of Nutrition Transition." Jianjun Zhang, Ishwori B. Dhakal, Zijn Zhao, et al. September 2012.
https://pubmed.ncbi.nlm.nih.gov/22357483/
4. PubMed, NIH, National Library of Medicine. "Nutritional Update for Physicians: Plant-Based Diets." Philip J. Tuso, Mohamed H. Ismail, Benjamin P. Ha, et al. Spring 2013.
https://pubmed.ncbi.nlm.nih.gov/23704846/
5. PMC, US National Library of Medicine, National Institutes of Health. "Epidemiology of Prostate Cancer." Prashanth Rawla. April 2019.
https://www.ncbi.nlm.nih.gov/pmc/articles/PMC6497009/#!po=4.60526
6. PubMed, NIH, National Library of Medicine. "Cancer Incidence in Japanese in Japan, Hawaii and Western United States." S. Tominaga. December 1985.
https://pubmed.ncbi.nlm.nih.gov/3834350/
7. World Health Organization. "Noncommunicable diseases." June 2018.
https://www.who.int/news-room/fact-sheets/detail/noncommunicable-diseases.

8. The New England Journal of Medicine. "Global Noncommunicable Diseases—Where Worlds Meet." K. M. Venkat Narayan, Mohammed K. Ali, Jeffrey P. Koplan. September 23, 2010.
https://www.nejm.org/doi/full/10.1056/NEJMp1002024
9. PubMed, NIH, National Library of Medicine. "Cardiovascular Effects of Androgen Deprivation Therapy for the Treatment of Prostate Cancer: ABCDE Steps to Reduce Cardiovascular Disease in Patients with Prostate Cancer." Nirmanmoh Bhatia, Marilia Santos, Lee W. Jones, et al. February 2016.
https://pubmed.ncbi.nlm.nih.gov/26831435/
10. PMC, US National Library of Medicine, National Institutes of Health. "What Do Prostate Cancer Patients Die Of?" Matias Riihimäki, Hauke Thomsen, Andreas Brandt, et al. January 2011.
https://www.ncbi.nlm.nih.gov/pmc/articles/PMC3228081/
11. British Journal of Cancer (BJC). "Cardiovascular disease risk and androgen deprivation therapy in patients with localized prostate cancer: a prospective cohort study." Reina Haque, Marianne UlcickasYood, Xiaoqing Xu, et al. October 2017.
https://www.nature.com/articles/bjc2017280#citeas

12. PubMed, NIH, National Library of Medicine. "Impact of Chronic Dietary Red Meat, White Meat, or Non-Meat Protein on Trimethylamine N-oxide Metabolism and Renal Excretion in Healthy Men and Women." Zeneng Wang, Nathalie Bergeron, Bruce S. Levison, et al. February 2019.
https://pubmed.ncbi.nlm.nih.gov/30535398/
13. American Institute for Cancer Research. "Food, Nutrition, Physical Activity, and the Prevention of Cancer: A Global Perspective." 2007.
https://b-ok.org/book/1214350/f6c0cb/
14. Harvard Health Publishing, Harvard Medical School. "Cutting red meat—for a longer life." June 2012.
https://www.health.harvard.edu/staying-healthy/cutting-red-meat-for-a-longer-life
15. PubMed, NIH, National Library of Medicine. "Association of Changes in Red Meat Consumption with Total and Cause Specific Mortality Among US Women and Men: Two Prospective Cohort Studies." Yan Zheng, Yanping Li, Ambika Satija, et al. June 2019.
https://pubmed.ncbi.nlm.nih.gov/31189526/
16. PMC, US National Library of Medicine, National Institutes of Health. "Meat intake and mortality: a prospective study of over half a million people." Rashmi Sinha, Amanda J. Cross, Barry I. Graubard, et al. March 2010.

https://www.ncbi.nlm.nih.gov/pmc/articles/PMC2803089/
17. PubMed, NIH, National Library of Medicine. "Reducing Meat Consumption Has Multiple Benefits for the World's Health." Barry M. Popkin. March 2009.
https://pubmed.ncbi.nlm.nih.gov/19307515/

Chapter 33

1. PMC, US National Library of Medicine, National Institutes of Health. "Insulin-like growth Factor-I and risk of differentiated thyroid carcinoma in the European Prospective Investigation into Cancer and Nutrition." Schmidt, Julie A., Naomi E. Allen, Martin Almquist, et al. March 2014.
https://www.ncbi.nlm.nih.gov/pmc/articles/PMC4046912/
2. PubMed, NIH, National Library of Medicine. "The Effect of Diet on Serum Insulin-Like Growth-Factor-I and Its Main Binding Proteins." N. E. Allen, P. N. Appleby, G. K. Davey, et al. 2002.
https://pubmed.ncbi.nlm.nih.gov/12484190/
3. PubMed, NIH, National Library of Medicine. "Hormones and Diet: Low Insulin-Like Growth Factor-I but Normal Bioavailable Androgens in Vegan Men." N. E. Allen, P. N. Appleby,

G. K. Davey, et al. 2000.
https://pubmed.ncbi.nlm.nih.gov/10883675/
4. Alternative Medicine Review. William B. Grant, PhD. "An Ecologic Study of Dietary Links to Prostate Cancer." 1999.
http://altmedrev.com/archive/publications/4/3/162.pdf
5. PubMed, NIH, National Library of Medicine. "Choline Intake and Risk of Lethal Prostate Cancer: Incidence and Survival." Erin L. Richman, Stacey A. Kenfield, Meir J. Stampfer, et al. October 2012.
https://pubmed.ncbi.nlm.nih.gov/22952174/
6. United States of America Dairy Industry, IUF Dairy Division. "Abstract—U.S. Dairy Industry." Business Wire (2011). "Research and Markets: The US Milk and Dairy Products Market Outlook to 2016-Introduction," USDA (2006) "Dairy Backgrounder," USDA (2010) "Overview of the United States Dairy Industry." et al. http://www.iuf.org/sites/cms.iuf.org/files/USA%20Dairy%20Industry.pdf
7. Alternative Medicine Review. William B. Grant, PhD. PubMed, NIH, National Library of Medicine. "An Ecologic Study of Dietary Links to Prostate Cancer." W. B. Grant. June 1999.
http://altmedrev.com/archive/publications/4/3/162.pdf

8. PubMed, NIH, National Library of Medicine. "Dairy Products, Calcium, Phosphorous, Vitamin D, and Risk of Prostate Cancer (Sweden)." J. M. Chan, E. Giovannucci, S. O. Andersson, et al. December 1998.
https://pubmed.ncbi.nlm.nih.gov/10189041/
9. PubMed, NIH, National Library of Medicine. "Dietary Patterns After Prostate Cancer Diagnosis in Relation to Disease—Specific and Total Mortality." Meng Yang, Stacey A. Kenfield, Erin L. VanBlarigan, et al. June 2015.
https://pubmed.ncbi.nlm.nih.gov/26031631/
10. PubMed, NIH, National Library of Medicine. "Dietary Correlates of Plasma Insulin-Like Growth Factor I and Insulin-Like Growth Factor Binding Protein 3 Concentrations." Michelle D. Holmes, Michael N. Pollak, Walter C. Willett, et al. September 2002.
https://pubmed.ncbi.nlm.nih.gov/12223429/
11. Journal of the American Dietetic Association. "Dietary Changes Favorably Affect Bone Remodeling in Older Adults." Robert P. Heaney, David A. McCarron, Bess Dawson-Hughes, et al. October 1999.
https://www.sciencedirect.com/science/article/abs/pii/S0002822399003028
12. PubMed, NIH, National Library of Medicine. "Hormones and Diet: Low Insulin-Like Growth Factor-I but Normal Bioavailable Androgens in Vegan Men." N. E. Allen, P. N. Appleby, G. K.

Davey, et al. July 2000.
https://pubmed.ncbi.nlm.nih.gov/10883675/
13. PubMed, NIH, National Library of Medicine. "Milk Consumption Is a Risk Factor for Prostate Cancer in Western Countries: Evidence from Cohort Studies." Li-Qiang Qin, Jia-Ying Xu, Pei-Yu "Wang, et al. 2007.
https://pubmed.ncbi.nlm.nih.gov/17704029/
14. PubMed, NIH, National Library of Medicine. "Milk Consumption Is a Risk Factor for Prostate Cancer: Meta-Analysis of Case-Control Studies." Li-Qiang Qin, Jia-Ying Xu, Pei-Yu Wang, et al. 2004.
https://pubmed.ncbi.nlm.nih.gov/15203374/
15. PubMed, NIH, National Library of Medicine. "A Prospective Study on Intake of Animal Products and Risk of Prostate Cancer." D. S. Michaud, K. Augustsson, E. B. Rimm, et al. August 2001.
https://pubmed.ncbi.nlm.nih.gov/11519764/
16. PubMed, NIH, National Library of Medicine. "A Prospective Study of Dietary Fat and Risk of Prostate Cancer." E. Giovannucci, E. B. Rimm, G. A. Colditz, et al. October 1993.
https://pubmed.ncbi.nlm.nih.gov/8105097/
17. Cancer Research United Kingdom Epidemiology Unit, University of Oxford. *Cancer Epidemiology, Biomarkers & Prevention.* "The Associations of Diet with Serum Insulin-Like Growth Factor I and Its Main Binding Proteins in 292 Women Meat-Eaters, Vegetarians, and Vegans."

Naomi E. Allen, Paul N. Appleby, Gwyneth K. Davey, et al. November 2002.
https://cebp.aacrjournals.org/content/cebp/11/11/1441.full.pdf

18. Elsevier, *Environmental Research.* "Carcinogenicity of consumption of red and processed meat: What about environmental contaminants?" José L. Domingo, Martí Nada. February 2016.
https://www.sciencedirect.com/science/article/abs/pii/S0013935115301596?via%3Dihub

19. PubMed, NIH, National Library of Medicine. "Diet, Androgens, Oxidative Stress, and Prostate Cancer Susceptibility." N. E. Fleshner, L. H. Klotz. December 1998.
https://pubmed.ncbi.nlm.nih.gov/10453275/

20. PubMed, NIH, National Library of Medicine. "Cancers Associated with High-Fat Diets." C. LaVecchia. 1992.
https://pubmed.ncbi.nlm.nih.gov/1616815/

21. PMC, US National Library of Medicine, National Institutes of Health. "Calorie restriction and cancer prevention: metabolic and molecular mechanisms." Valter D. Longo, Luigi Fontana. January 2010.
https://www.ncbi.nlm.nih.gov/pmc/articles/PMC2829867/

22. PMC, US National Library of Medicine, National Institutes of Health. "Egg, red meat, and poultry intake and risk of lethal prostate cancer in the prostate-specific antigen-era: incidence

and survival." Erin L. Richman, Stacey A. Kenfield, Meir J. Stampfer, et al. September 2011.
https://www.ncbi.nlm.nih.gov/pmc/articles/PMC3232297/

23. PubMed, NIH, National Library of Medicine. "One-carbon Metabolism and Prostate Cancer Risk: Prospective Investigation of Seven Circulating B Vitamins and Metabolites." Mattias Johansson, Bethany Van Guelpen, Stein Emil Vollset, et al. May 2009.
https://pubmed.ncbi.nlm.nih.gov/19423531/

24. Cleveland Heart Lab. "Choline, TMAO, and Heart Health." May 2017.
https://www.clevelandheartlab.com/blog/choline-tmao-heart-health/.

25. PMC, US National Library of Medicine, National Institutes of Health. "Choline intake and risk of lethal prostate cancer: incidence and survival." Erin L. Richman, Stacey A. Kenfield, Meir J. Stampfer, et al. September 2012.
https://www.ncbi.nlm.nih.gov/pmc/articles/PMC3441112/

26. PMC, US National Library of Medicine, National Institutes of Health. "Intakes of meat, fish, poultry, and eggs, and risk of prostate cancer progression." (Abstract's Results). December 2009.
https://www.ncbi.nlm.nih.gov/pmc/articles/PMC3132069/

27. Journal of Exposure Science & Environmental Epidemiology. "U.S. dietary exposures to heterocyclic amines." P. Armitage and R. Doll, "A two-stage theory of carcinogenesis in relation to the age distribution of human cancer"; K. Augustsson, K. Skog, M. Jagerstad, et all., "Dietary heterocyclic amines and cancer of the colon, rectum, bladder, and kidney: a population based study."; K. Agustsson, K. Skog, M. Jagerstad, et al., "Assessment of the human exposure to heterocyclic amines"; et al. July 2001.
https://www.nature.com/articles/7500158

28. PMC, US National Library of Medicine, National Institutes of Health. "Intakes of meat, fish, poultry, and eggs and risk of prostate cancer progression." (Results below "Statistical methods.") December 2009.
https://www.ncbi.nlm.nih.gov/pmc/articles/PMC3132069/

29. PMC, US National Library of Medicine, National Institutes of Health. Oxford Journals, American Journal of Epidemiology. "Serum Phospholipid Fatty Acids and Prostate Cancer Risk: Results from the Prostate Cancer Prevention Trial." Theodore M. Brasky, Cathee Till, Emily White, et al. April 2011.
https://www.ncbi.nlm.nih.gov/pmc/articles/PMC3145396/

30. JAMA Network (JAMA Cardiology). "Associations of Omega-3 Fatty Acid Supplement Use

with Cardiovascular Disease Risks: Meta-analysis of 10 Trials Involving 77,917 Individuals." Theingi Aung, Jim Halsey, Daan Kromhout, et al. March 2018.
https://jamanetwork.com/journals/jamacardiology/fullarticle/2670752

31. PMC, US National Library of Medicine, National Institutes of Health. "Serum Phospholipid Fatty Acids and Prostate Cancer Risk: Results from the Prostate Cancer Prevention Trial." Theodore M. Brasky, Cathee Till, Emily White, et al. April 2011.
https://www.ncbi.nlm.nih.gov/pmc/articles/PMC3145396/

32. PMC, US National Library of Medicine, National Institutes of Health. "Omega-3 Fatty Acids and Cardiovascular Disease: Are There Benefits?" Kate J. Bowen, William S. Harris, and Penny M. Kris-Etherton. October 2016.
https://www.ncbi.nlm.nih.gov/pmc/articles/PMC5067287/

33. PubMed, NIH, National Library of Medicine. "Fatty Fish Consumption and Risk of Prostate Cancer." P. Terry, P. Lichtenstein, M. Feychting, et al. June 2001.
https://pubmed.ncbi.nlm.nih.gov/11403817/

34. PMC, US National Library of Medicine, National Institutes of Health. "A 22-year prospective study of fish intake in relation to prostate cancer incidence and mortality." Jorge

E. Chavarro, Meir J. Stampfer, Megan N. Hall, et al. March 2010.
https://www.ncbi.nlm.nih.gov/pmc/articles/PMC2843087/.

35. BJC (British Journal of Cancer). Epidemiology. "Omega-3, omega-6 and total dietary polyunsaturated fat on cancer incidence: systematic review and meta-analysis of randomised trials." Sarah Hanson, Gabrielle Thorpe, Lauren Winstanley, et al. February 2020.
https://www.bbcgoodfood.com/sites/default/files/editor_files/2020/02/41416_2020_761_online pdf_2_0.pdf

37. Food and Agriculture Organization. "Globefish -Information and Analysis on World Fish Trade (Farmed fish: a major provider or a major consumer of omega-3 oils?)" Jogeir Toppe.
http://www.fao.org/in-action/globefish/fishery-information/resource-detail/en/c/338773/.

38. World Health Organization. "Dioxins and their effects on human health." October 2016.
https://www.who.int/news-room/fact-sheets/detail/dioxins-and-their-effects-on-human-health

39. A joint project by the Universities of Oregon State, Cornell, Delaware, et al. "Overview of the U.S. Seafood Supply."
https://www.seafoodhealthfacts.org/seafood-choices/overview-us-seafood-supply

40. Healthline. "Wild vs Farmed Salmon: Which Type of Salmon Is Healthier?" https://www.healthline.com/nutrition/wild-vs-farmed-salmon
41. Jama Network. "Effect of Omega-3 Fatty Acids, Lutein/Zeaxanthin, or Other Nutrient Supplementation on Cognitive Function The AREDS2 Randomized Clinical Trial." Emily Y. Chew, Traci E. Clemons, Elvira Agrón. August 2015. https://jamanetwork.com/journals/jama/fullarticle/2429713
42. PMC, US National Library of Medicine, National Institutes of Health. "Type of Vegetarian Diet, Body Weight, and Prevalence of Type 2 Diabetes." Serena Tonstad, Terry Butler, Ru Yan, et al. May 2009. https://www.ncbi.nlm.nih.gov/pmc/articles/PMC2671114/
43. AAAS (American Association for the Advancement of Science). "The economics of fishing the high seas." Enric Sala, Juan Mayorga, Christopher Costello, et al. June 2018. https://advances.sciencemag.org/content/4/6/eaat2504
44. PubMed, NIH, National Library of Medicine. "Fish Consumption, omega-3 Fatty Acids and the Mediterranean Diet." R. García-Closas, L. Serra-Majem, R. Segura. September 1993. https://pubmed.ncbi.nlm.nih.gov/8269907/

45. U. S. Preventive Services Task Force. "Vitamin Supplementation to Prevent Cancer and CVD: Preventive Medication." R. L. Bailey, J. J. Gahche, C. V. Lentino, et al. September 2014. https://www.uspreventiveservicestaskforce.org/uspstf/document/RecommendationStatementFinal/vitamin-supplementation-to-prevent-cancer-and-cvd-counseling

Chapter 34

1. PubMed, NIH, National Library of Medicine. "Colorectal Cancer and the Intake of Nutrients: Oligosaccharides Are a Risk Factor, Fats Are Not. A Case-Control Study in Belgium." A. J. Tuyns, M. Haelterman, R. Kaaks. 1987. https://pubmed.ncbi.nlm.nih.gov/2829139/
2. PubMed, NIH, National Library of Medicine. "Dietary Polyunsaturated Fat Versus Saturated Fat in Relation to Mammary Carcinogenesis." K. K. Carroll, G. J. Hopkins. February 1979. https://pubmed.ncbi.nlm.nih.gov/106196/
3. PubMed, NIH, National Library of Medicine. "Moderate Alcohol Consumption and the Risk of Breast Cancer." W. C. Willett, M. J. Stampfer, G. A. Colditz, et al. May 1987. https://pubmed.ncbi.nlm.nih.gov/3574368/
4. PubMed, NIH, National Library of Medicine. "Pilot Study of Dietary Fat Restriction and

Flaxseed Supplementation in Men with Prostate Cancer Before Surgery: Exploring the Effects on Hormonal Levels, Prostate-Specific Antigen, and Histopathologic Features." W. Demark-Wahnefried, D. T. Price, T. J. Polascik, et al. July 2001.
https://pubmed.ncbi.nlm.nih.gov/11445478/
5. PubMed, NIH, National Library of Medicine. "The Postprandial Effect of Components of the Mediterranean Diet on Endothelial Function." R. A. Vogel, M. C. Corretti, G. D. Plotnick. November 2000.
https://pubmed.ncbi.nlm.nih.gov/11079642/

Chapter 35

1. PubMed, NIH, National Library of Medicine. "Are Strict Vegetarians Protected Against Pros Cancer?" Yessenia Tantamango-Bartley, Synnove F. Knutsen, Raymond Knutsen, et al. January 2016.
https://www.ncbi.nlm.nih.gov/pubmed/26561618/
2. PubMed, NIH, National Library of Medicine. "Position of the Academy of Nutrition and Dietetics: Vegetarian Diets." Vesanto Melina, Winston Craig, Susan Levin. December 2016.
https://pubmed.ncbi.nlm.nih.gov/27886704/.
3. World Health Organization. "Healthy Diet." L. Hooper, A. Abdelhamid, D. Bunn, et al. October 2018.

https://www.who.int/news-room/fact-sheets/detail/healthy-diet.

4. PubMed, NIH, National Library of Medicine. "Current Protein Intake in America: Analysis of the National Health and Nutrition Examination Survey, 2003-2004." Victor L. Fulgoni 3rd. May 2008.
https://pubmed.ncbi.nlm.nih.gov/18469286/

5. The Journal of Nutrition (Oxford Academic). "Soybean Phytochemicals Inhibit the Growth of Transplantable Human Prostate Carcinoma and Tumor Angiogenesis in Mice." Jin-Rong Zhou, Eric T. Gugger, Toshihide Tanaka, et al. September 1999.
https://academic.oup.com/jn/article/129/9/1628/4721938

6. AACR Publications (American Association for Cancer Research). "Soy Food Consumption and Breast Cancer Prognosis." Bette J. Caan, Loki Natarajan, Barbara Parker, et al. May 2011.
https://cebp.aacrjournals.org/content/20/5/854

7. PubMed, NIH, National Library of Medicine. "Effect of Soy Isoflavones on Breast Cancer Recurrence and Death for Patients Receiving Adjuvant Endocrine Therapy." Xinmei Kang, Qingyuan Zhang, Shuhuai Wang, et al. November 2010.
https://pubmed.ncbi.nlm.nih.gov/20956506/

8. PubMed, NIH, National Library of Medicine. "Effect of soy isoflavones on breast cancer recurrence and death for patients receiving adjuvant endocrine therapy." Xinmei Kang, Quigyuan Ahang, Shuhuai Wang, et. al. November 2010.
https://pubmed.ncbi.nlm.nih.gov/20956506/.
9. Springer. "Soy isoflavones consumption and risk of breast cancer incidence or recurrence: a meta-analysis of prospective studies." Jia-Yi Dong and Li-Qiang Qin. November 2010.
https://link.springer.com/article/10.1007%2Fs10549-010-1270-8#citeas
10. U. S. Department of Agriculture. (Food Surveys Research Group.) "Fiber intake of the U.S. population: What We Eat in America, NHANES 2009-2010." M. Katherine Hoy, Rd. Goldman, Joseph D. Goldman. September 2014.
https://www.ars.usda.gov/ARSUserFiles/80400530/pdf/DBrief/12_fiber_intake_0910.pdf
11. PubMed, NIH, National Library of Medicine. "Sodium Butyrate Promotes Apoptosis in Breast Cancer Cells Through Reactive Oxygen Species (ROS) Formation and Mitochondrial Impairment." Vahid Salimi, Zahra Shahsavari, Banafsheh Safizadeh, et al. November 2017.
https://pubmed.ncbi.nlm.nih.gov/29096636/.

Chapter 36

1. PubMed, NIH, National Library of Medicine. "Follow-up of Water-Only Fasting and an Exclusively Plant Food Diet in the Management of Stage IIIa, Low-Grade Follicular Lymphoma." Toshia R. Myers, Mary Zittel, Alan C. Goldhamer. August 2018.
https://pubmed.ncbi.nlm.nih.gov/30093470/
2. PMC, US National Library of Medicine, National Institutes of Health. "Protein Quantity and Source, Fasting-Mimicking Diets, and Longevity." Sebastian Brandhorst and Valter D. Longo. November 2019.
https://www.ncbi.nlm.nih.gov/pmc/articles/PMC6855936/
3. PMC, US National Library of Medicine, National Institutes of Health. "Nutrient Restriction and Radiation Therapy for Cancer Treatment: When Less Is More: Nutrient Restriction and Radiation Therapy for Cancer Treatment: When Less Is More." Colin E. Champ, Renato Baserga, Mark V. Mishra, et al. January 2013.
https://www.ncbi.nlm.nih.gov/pmc/articles/PMC3556263/
4. USC News (University of Southern California). "Fasting weakens cancer in mice." Carl Marziali. February 2012.
https://news.usc.edu/29428/fasting-weakens-cancer-in-mice/

5. PubMed, NIH, National Library of Medicine. "Effects of Short-Term Fasting on Cancer Treatment." Stefanie de Groot, Hanno Pijl, Jacobus J. M. van der Hoeven, et al. May 2019.
https://pubmed.ncbi.nlm.nih.gov/31113478/
6. PubMed, NIH, National Library of Medicine. (Clinical Trials.gov) "Fasting and Nutritional Therapy in Patients with Advanced Metastatic Prostate Cancer." Andreas Michalsen, Charite University, Berlin, Germany. March 2016 (Updated February 2020).
https://clinicaltrials.gov/ct2/show/NCT02710721

ABOUT THE AUTHOR

Bruce Mylrea lives and travels full-time with his wife Mindy in their 32-foot fruit and vegetable covered RV. They travel across North America providing lectures and education on whole-food, plant-based nutrition.

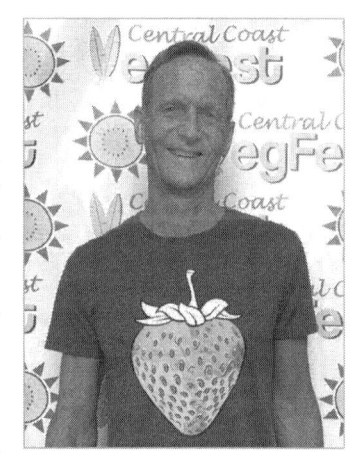

Bruce is a certified (AFPA) holistic nutritional counselor and a proud graduate of the e-Cornell Plant-Based Nutrition Certification Program. He spends hours each day researching evidence-based nutrition with a focus on cancer.

Bruce is also an award-winning speaker and educator at fitness and wellness conferences around the world. Bruce and Mindy created the nine hour One Day to Wellness certification program and have presented it to thousands of people around the world. Bruce and Mindy also teach oil-free plant-based cooking classes as part of their non-profit mission. They are a non-profit 501(c)3 organization.

ALSO AVAILABLE ON AMAZON

MINDY'S BOOK

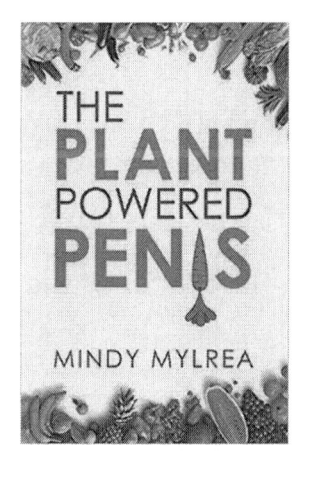

THE PLANT POWERED PENIS

MINDY MYLREA

https://www.amazon.com/Plant-Powered-Penis-Mindy-Mylrea/dp/B086PNZM5G/ref=sr_1_2?dchild=1&keywords=the+plant+powered+penis&qid=1596561239&sr=8-2

REVIEWS

Foods have powerful effects on health—they can help you lose weight, lower cholesterol, and even reduce your cancer risk. But there is one benefit you might not have anticipated, and that is their effect on your sex life.

Give it a try, and you'll see what I mean. This engaging book brings you the information you need, along with delicious recipes to put it to work.

> Neal D. Barnard, MD
> Adjunct Professor
> George Washington University School of Medicine
> President, Physicians Committee

This entertaining book engages readers with the science and research of eating a whole food, plant-based diet without added oil and also with Mindy's personal experience of how plant-based nutrition plays an important role in a healthy marriage/partnership and health overall.

> John McDougall, MD
> Founder of the McDougall Program
> Best-selling author—The Starch Solution

IT'S ABOUT TIME for this book to come out! I've health coached hundreds of men over a decade now, and they need this NOW more than ever! This quick, easy-to-read guide will give you all the "action" steps you need to take your health back into your own hands! Thank you, Mindy, for bringing this book to life! Can't wait to give them out as Holiday Gifts!

> Michelle Joy Kramer
> Board Certified Health Coach,
> CHHC, AADP

Also Available on Amazon - Mindy's Book - Reviews

Playful and sexy in its delivery, the information Mylrea shares is health positive regardless of your genitalia. Whether you choose to go fully vegan or not, a plant-based diet is clearly associated with enhanced wellbeing, reducing the risk of chronic illness such as obesity, diabetes, heart disease, and cancer. Helpful motivating tips and enticing recipes provide practical resources to encourage the adoption of improved nutrition for a healthier lifestyle.

> Donald I. Abrams, MD, Integrative Oncologist,
> UCSF Osher Center for Integrative Medicine
> Professor of Clinical Medicine,
> University of California San Francisco

Books on sex and diet are among the most popular books read today. This is a book about both. It is a must-read for every man that wants to maintain a healthy body and a healthy sex life throughout his life. This book demonstrates how the power of plant-based nutrition can help men maintain a healthy sex life throughout life.

> John Westerdahl, PhD, MPH, RDN, FAND
> Radio Talk Show Host
> Past Chair, Vegetarian Nutrition
> Dietetic Practice Group of the
> Academy of Nutrition and Dietetics

Vegan is the new viagra! In this delightful book you'll learn that what's good for your heart is good for all of your organs. Why take a blue pill when you can eat a green leaf?

Chef AJ
Author: *The Secrets To Ultimate Weight Loss*

What a great read. Informative, hopeful, hilarious, and full of tangible action items to include right away to support optimal health. The lessons in this book will help every gender and every cell and organ in your body."

— Ocean Robbins, Co-founder
Food Revolution Network
Author, 31-Day Food Revolution